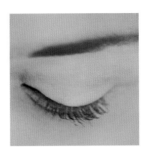

Ann Redfearn

Migraine

Take control of your health naturally

D1213956

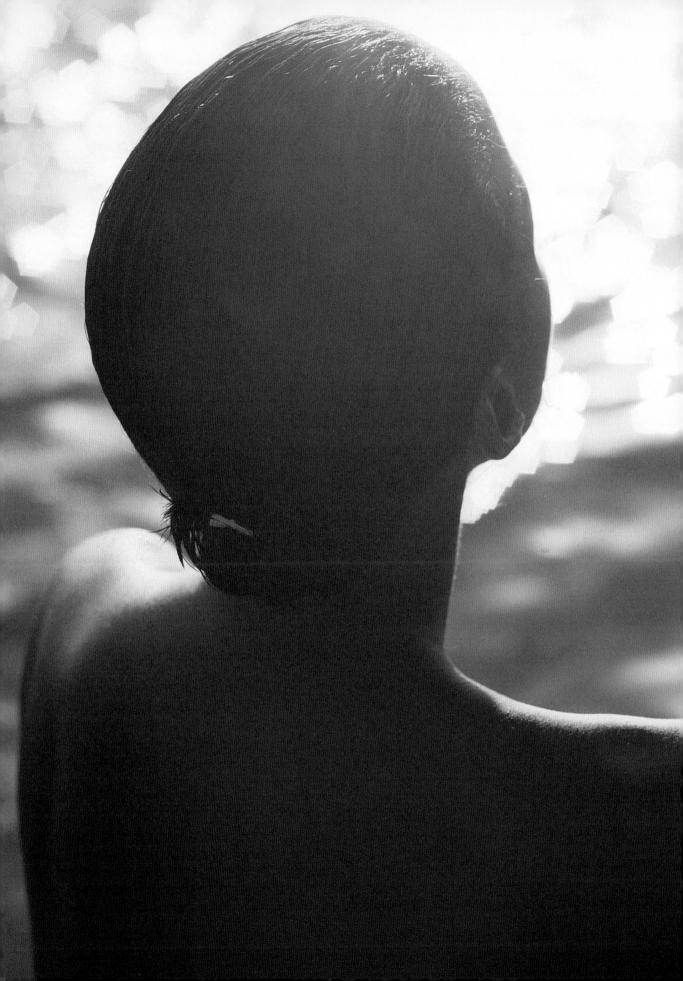

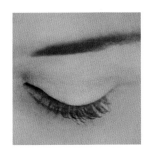

Ann Redfearn

Migraine

Take control of your health naturally

Gaia Books

Project Editor Kelly Thompson
Design Phil Gamble
Photography Ruth Jenkinson, Dave King,
            Paul Forrester, Gus Filgate
Direction Jo Godfrey Wood, Patrick Nugent

First published in 2005 in the United Kingdom by:
Gaia Books, an imprint of Octopus Publishing Group Ltd
2–4 Heron Quays, Canary Wharf, London E14 4JP

Text © Ann Redfearn 2005
Illustrations and compilation © Gaia Books 2005

A CIP catalogue record for this book is available from the British
library:

ISBN: 1-85675-233-X

Distributed in the United States and Canada by
Sterling Publishing Co., Inc., 387 Park Avenue South, New York, NY 10016–8810

Manufactured in China

10 9 8 7 6 5 4 3 2 1

Author photograph: Peter Carrick

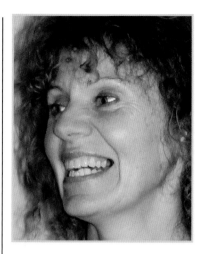

Author: Ann Redfearn BSY (DS, Arom, Col)

Ann is a qualified tai chi and kai men (Chinese Yoga) instructor, who has been studying and teaching for seventeen years. She is also a qualified aroma-therapist, colour therapist, holistic diagnostician, and feng shui practitioner. Her experience has led to an awareness of and sensitivity to the human energy field and through this she has developed a range of varying natural healing techniques – in the knowledge that different people have different needs, changing and developing over time. To share her enriching experience of healing energy, Ann has recently started writing books offering holistic advice and self-help techniques, with the hope that a wider audience might benefit as much as she, her friends, her family, and her clients have done over the years.

Contents

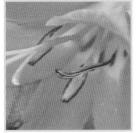

Disclaimer

The information and exercises given within this book are in no way intended to replace professional medical advice. Neither the author nor the publishers shall be liable or responsible for any loss, injury, or damage allegedly arising from any information or suggestion in this book.

Introduction

Migraine is a very distressing condition for which there is, as yet, no cure in Western medical terms. There are many drugs available to help manage the pain and lessen the severity of an attack, but nothing to help with initial prevention.

A migraine differs from a normal headache in that it is characterized by a deep throbbing and highly debilitating pain, usually – but not always – on one side of the head. It may begin with a distortion in the vision, such as flashing lights, or a zig zag or tunnel effect in the line of vision. As the head pain worsens, it is often accompanied by nausea and, in severe cases, vomiting. The pain in the head may become extremely severe, with sensitivity to bright lights and noise. And a lack of concentration also seems to form part of the picture, as

does a general feeling of being "oversensitive". These symptoms don't often last for more than a day, but can leave the sufferer feeling weakened and exhausted for several days afterwards. Attacks may only come once in a while or may be fairly regular. Every individual's experience of them is slightly different.

Who gets migraines and why?

According to the World Health Organisation (WHO) figures, more than ten percent of the Western population suffer from migraines. These can start at any age, although they often start in the teens and have been known to start even younger.

Statistically, nearly three times as many women as men suffer from migraine attacks, and it is therefore thought that there may, in some instances, be a link with the menstrual cycle. However, migraines can also be brought on by many other

factors, such as eye strain, sinus congestion, muscular tension, fatigue, lack of fresh air, lack of exercise, excessive exercise, hunger, dehydration, stress, or unresolved emotions (see box right). Headaches and migraines can also accompany back or neck problems, which, in some cases, are posture-related.

Those who frequently suffer from migraine or severe headaches are often aware that something in particular "triggers" the attack, or that their migraines occur for a combination of reasons. Perhaps, if you're not aware of any specific cause or causes, this book will help you to develop a deeper understanding of your condition and to identify your own personal triggers. It may be underlying tension and anxiety, a particular food, or certain external conditions, such as flickering lights, noise, or pollution. A "liverish" migraine, for example – which is often accompanied by feelings of nausea or actual vomiting – can be brought on by an excess

Symptoms

★ *Deep, throbbing pain – often on one side of the head only*
★ *Distorted vision or flashing lights*
★ *Nausea or vomiting*
★ *Extreme sensitivity to light and noise*
★ *Lack of ability to focus or concentrate*

A STRESSFUL LIFESTYLE
It now seems that migraine is somehow linked to the fast pace of life so many of us now lead. A wide variety of trigger factors (see box right) also contribute.

of fatty foods, which affect the liver and gall bladder, leading to a congested, bilious headache.

Recent research, however, has found that the number of people suffering from migraines is very much on the increase – so much so that it has been named among the world's top twenty most disabling conditions by the World Health Organisation. This rising frequency of migraines would suggest that they may be in some way linked to the increasingly hectic, pressurized, and stressful lives that we often feel compelled to live in modern society.

The majority of people in today's society are now very far removed from nature and its cycles. Although we are not always aware of it, our bodies can find it very hard to maintain health and balance in this almost entirely man-made environment, being cut off from the natural cycle of the seasons – varying light and darkness, and natural fluctuations in temperature. There are often no natural breaks in our 24/7 buzz, with a mad dash to maintain constant activity, whether at work, commuting, socializing, or at home. Many peoples' leisure time even involves excessive use of flickering TV or computer screens, or taking exercise in controlled,

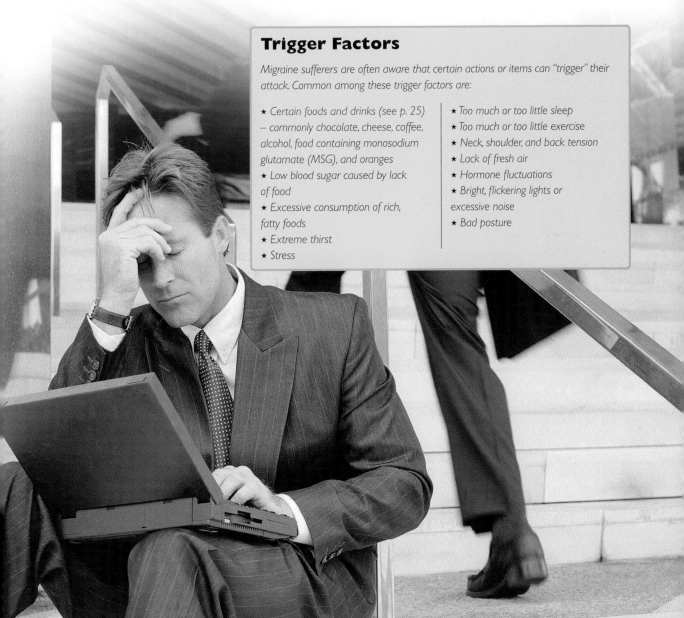

Trigger Factors

Migraine sufferers are often aware that certain actions or items can "trigger" their attack. Common among these trigger factors are:

★ Certain foods and drinks (see p. 25) – commonly chocolate, cheese, coffee, alcohol, food containing monosodium glutamate (MSG), and oranges
★ Low blood sugar caused by lack of food
★ Excessive consumption of rich, fatty foods
★ Extreme thirst
★ Stress

★ Too much or too little sleep
★ Too much or too little exercise
★ Neck, shoulder, and back tension
★ Lack of fresh air
★ Hormone fluctuations
★ Bright, flickering lights or excessive noise
★ Bad posture

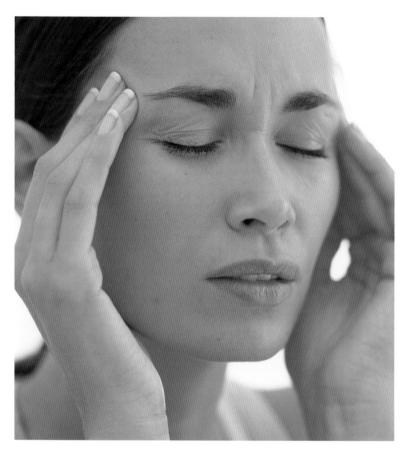

FEELING THE STRAIN
Migraine attacks often come about at times of extreme pressure and/or tiredness as a result of our ever-faster pace of life and the many demands that we – and others – place on ourselves.

when faced with pain (such as during a migraine attack), "Why me?" or "What have I done to deserve this?". These are questions of the spirit, to which science has yet to provide cohesive answers, if it ever can.

So, although we can often be shown in incredible detail what has "gone wrong" with our bodies in physical terms, and we can now benefit from quite a phenomenal degree of help on this level, we may well find ourselves asking what has caused these "malfunctions" in our bodies in the first place?

There is a strong school of thought that now believes our physical sickness, whether in the form of migraines or anything else, is a mirror-image of any emotional sickness that lies within. This belief is based upon the workings of the human energy field. Our energy field – or aura, as it is sometimes known – is made up, in part, of an extraordinarily complicated network of emotions, personal beliefs, and entrenched thought patterns. This is where we hold all our life experiences – both good and bad – until such a time as they are healed, defused, or let go of. This intricate energy network has a direct influence on the physical body, via the pathways

artificial surroundings, with electric lighting, piped music, air-conditioning and/or heating, and electronic exercise equipment. Such constant stimuli can result in stress and tension, giving rise to symptoms such as migraines and headaches. Another cause of these tension headaches is the apparent need to be "on call" all the time. The society in which we live has conditioned us to expect ourselves – and others – to be as "instant" as the technology that now drives it. We are not, however, "instant" beings, but have needs and requirements of our own, which frequently get

dismissed or overlooked, to the detriment of our health. These needs include a fresh, healthy, balanced diet, rest, relaxation, and general enjoyment of life.

Time to look within

We live in an age in which science seeks to provide the answers to everything. This has enabled society to make enormous leaps forward in terms of health, communication, and travel. Although many answers that we seek can be found at the press of a button, there are others that remain shrouded in mystery. There aren't many of us, for example, who have not asked, of energy called meridian lines (see p. 76–77) and the energy centres called chakras (see pp. 114–117). These give and receive information – in the form of thoughts, feelings, and memories – between the energetic field (our invisible body) and the physical body through which we directly experience life (our visible body).

As we go through life, we develop ways of coping with certain situations and reacting to stressful or threatening scenarios. We are largely creatures of habit, so become used to behaving or responding in ways that are familiar to us, and which, although they may have served us in the past, are no longer necessarily good for our health. For example, we may get used to swallowing our anger or to dismissing our needs as being less important than the needs of those around us. Perhaps we feel overly responsible for other people, not really trusting them to be able to sort out the ups and downs of their own lives, or we might habitually fret over the details of life, eating ourselves away with stresses and worries. Or we may have a particularly short fuse and "blow" at the slightest provocation, believing that life is somehow against us.

COMING TO TERMS

Letting go of stress and performing relaxation strategies can help you change your attitude to your self, your life, and the energy that is creating ill health in you.

Work and research in this field has led to the conclusion that illnesses, including migraines, have a certain "belief structure" that helps to form the cause of the sickness. Ill health develops in the energy field – and is present "energetically" – before we experience any actual physical symptoms. We are now aware, for example, that migraine attacks are often closely linked with unresolved feelings such as anger, frustration, and injustice – the feeling that life's not heading where you had been hoping or that "life's not fair!". See pp. 12–21 for further details on exploring and coming to terms with such emotions so that you can release yourself from any negative cycle into which you may have fallen.

A brief word about chi

You will become familiar with the word "chi" as you work through this book, because it is the energy upon which most of the self-healing methods are based. Chi is the word used by Chinese health practitioners to describe the life force within us – the subtle energy that pervades all living things and exists in a constant state of flow, breathing life into everything. It could be thought of as the "spirit of life".

It is felt that when the flow of chi is disrupted, illness of some form is experienced, whether physical, mental, emotional, or spiritual. Migraine can be an indication of imbalance in any or all of these areas. Good health, on the other hand, is when there is a perfectly

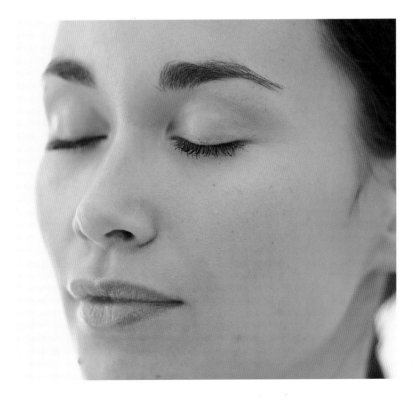

balanced flow of chi, unifying mind and body with universal energy. The stronger the overall flow of chi in a person, the healthier they are and the more resistant they tend to be to physical disorders such as migraines.

In Ancient China, doctors used to be employed full-time to keep their clients "in full balance" and therefore in good health – rather than to cure them once illness had already set in. Illness was therefore seen as a failure on the part of the physician, and payment at these times was withheld.

How to help yourself

There are many simple, but extremely effective, natural self-help techniques that you can try in order to restore both your body's life balance and energy balance and to bring about relief from painful conditions such as migraines – from altering your diet, to introducing some gentle exercise into your daily life, to making regular massage part of your routine, to dealing with unresolved emotions, to tuning into the healing power of colour, to simply learning to relax more. With this in mind, I have put together the suggestions in this book, so read on to find out how you can help yourself move toward a healthier, migraine-free existence.

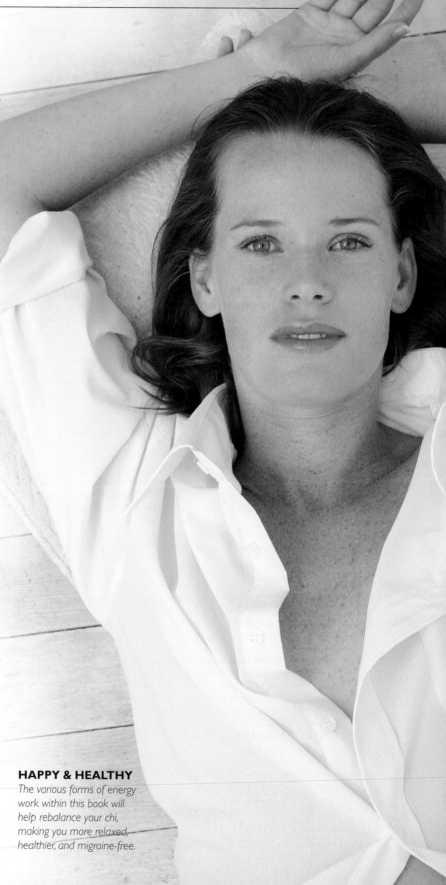

HAPPY & HEALTHY
The various forms of energy work within this book will help rebalance your chi, making you more relaxed, healthier, and migraine-free.

How to use
this book

This book contains a wide range of self-help methods that will help bring relief from migraines and severe headaches. They encompass a broad spectrum of natural methods, including dietary and exercise suggestions, and massage and relaxation techniques.

The self-help exercises suggested should not only lessen the frequency and severity of your migraines, but should also bring about improved general well-being and an increase in overall energy and vitality, as they teach you to relax and generally look after yourself more, thus restoring balance to your body's life force. Most importantly, however, they should help you release yourself from the feeling of frustration and imprisonment brought about by your regular bouts of pain and discomfort.

I recently used this programme to help my teenage daughter, who was suffering from frequent migraine attacks. Her discomfort was so severe that she would perspire from sheer pain, and any attempt to take medication would make her vomit. At the time, we were extremely distressed, but since I applied the methods within this book,

she has not had a single migraine. In her words, "It works!".

You can simply dip in and out of the suggestions, putting together a personal pick-and-mix, or you can progress logically through all the ideas – the choice is yours. One day you might feel like exploring your emotions, the next you might be in the mood to use aromatic oils, and the next you might prefer to treat yourself to a gentle meridian massage or indulge in a colour visualization. And do not worry: the exercises and techniques are all straight-forward and easy to follow, so should not be difficult for you to integrate into your daily life – even if you are already starting to feel the debilitating pain of a migraine coming on. Many of them simply teach the mind and body the art of relaxation.

All the techniques described should actively help in prevent-

ing the onset of a headache or migraine attack, or in reducing their severity or frequency, so it is up to you to experiment to find which ones work best for you. I found the following combination of treatments extremely successful for treating my own daughter's migraines over a period of just two weeks: the Pain Wizard herbal tea (see p. 56) twice daily, a ginger compress twice daily on her liver area (see pp. 58–59), the "Joy of Life" breathing exercise every morning and evening (see pp. 68–69), and the simple meridian massage techniques twice daily (pp. 78–81). Her increasingly frequent migraine attacks simply disappeared.

The art of healthy – and migraine-free – living could be viewed as the art of choice. And picking up this book and following the techniques within it means you have already made your first positive choice to build or rebuild healthy habits, which will, over time, increase the harmonious flow of healthy chi, thus reducing, and eventually eliminating, migraines.

It is advisable, however, to consult your doctor before trying any of the exercises if you are pregnant, or if you are in any doubt about the suitability of these techniques for you.

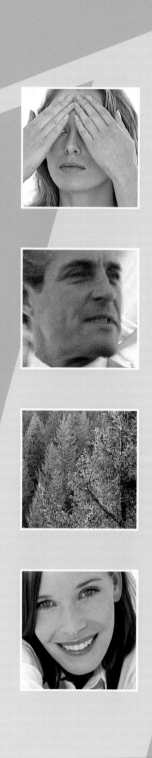

Chapter One

Exploring your
EMOTIONS

Through our feelings,

we know one another

And can, just for a fleeting moment,

Touch each other's worlds

The power of emotions

Migraines can often be the physical result of a negative emotional pattern or underlying emotional problem – even one of which you are initially unaware. It is therefore useful to take an honest look within yourself for a simple "cure".

It is useful to observe your thought patterns, your habitual responses to certain situations, and any recurring negative feelings that you experience. Then think about how these might relate to the timing of your migraine attacks.

Keeping a diary of the circumstances and feelings leading up to your attacks is a good idea as it might enable you to more easily see patterns emerging. You may discover – much to your surprise – that your migraines "happen" to coincide with times of extreme anger, resentment, frustration, or stress. Or you may find that they only occur when you have been letting feelings like this build up over long periods of time by repressing them. Alternatively, your headaches may be linked to feelings of inadequacy arising from fear of expressing opinions, of moving forward in life, or of trusting your intuition. Or they may be linked to feelings of "holding back" or of somehow being stifled, which can also cause tension in the neck and shoulders.

Body talk

When you really think about it, it's very natural that your body has a bad reaction to such negativity, as it's your body, let's not forget, that has to carry it all around on a daily basis. These extreme emotions are a sign, from a holistic perspective, that

The Emotions of the Organs

Chinese healing philosophy believes that each of the body's main five organs are related to specific emotions, which manifest themselves positively when the area is in balance, and negatively, causing problems like migraines, when it is out of balance.

Major Organ	Positive Emotions	Negative Emotions
Heart	Love, joy, sharing	Resentment, jealousy, hatred
Stomach	Nurturing, contentment	Anxiety
Lungs	Courage, resourcefulness	Depression, grief
Kidneys	Kindness	Fear
Liver	Gentleness	Anger

STRESS MANAGEMENT
It is extremely useful to be able to view our daily stress as no more than an emotional response to external circumstances, as this implies an element of choice – and therefore control – over what happens to us.

you are in a state of imbalance. And as you're not tuning into the subtle, energetic signs about the need to slow down, switch off, or calm down in order to restore balance, your body has to do something more drastic – and more physical – to which you will pay attention: pain! We are all familiar with how emotional feelings can affect the body. A simple example is how when we're feeling nervous we have to keep dashing to the loo, or when we feel angry our face becomes flushed and our pulse speeds up. In the case of migraines, the intense heat produced by the swirling emotions in the energetic field result in an implosion of pain in the head.

Dealing with stress

Stress is something that we all experience in our lives in some form or other. It's just that different people can deal with it on very different levels. The fact that stress may be at the root of your migraines in no way implies, however, that you are to blame for your illness. Instead, it serves as a pointer to the emotional issues that may need addressing.

The first step in resolving any emotional issues, or patterns, is to recognize that they are there. The next step is to find ways of breaking the habits that have become destructive enough to

cause your migraines. You may realize, for example, that it's better to tackle tough issues as they arise, rather than letting them build up into an inevitable volcano. Or you may need to deal with problems calmly, rather than trying to ignore them until they are so unbearable that you either erupt or have an internal crisis.

If your migraine attacks seem stress-related, then simply starting to alter your usual emotional reaction to stressful events will set you on the path to health. Several helpful ways of beginning to do this are offered on the following pages.

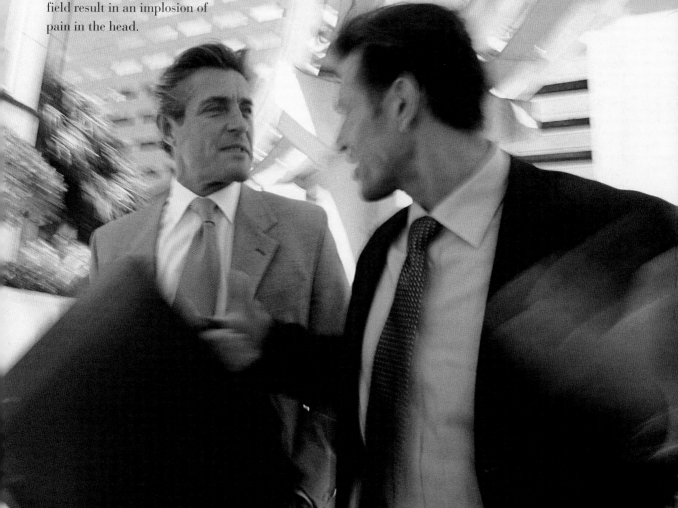

Still the *mind*

The arts of reflection, contemplation, and meditation (see also pages 60–73) are very useful for untangling webs of distressing emotions and thus alleviating migraines, as they can lead to increased clarity, allowing you to view problems as positive challenges.

If you can learn to still the mind for long enough to question the events leading up to your migraines, and if you get into the habit of keeping a note of what you discover, you can get a little closer to understanding how your mind and body operate.

Perhaps you need to learn to speak up for yourself, instead of trying to swallow and suppress difficult feelings. Or maybe you need to learn to discharge unreasoned anger in a less destructive way, through something like vigorous exercise, or simply climbing a hill and yelling into the wind!

A very effective way to train thoughts and emotions, encouraging them to become calmer and clearer, is to practise regular concentration or contemplation techniques. The suggestions on the following pages are all exercises for the mind.

Become a Calm Self-Observer

Try to look at every situation you are facing in terms of "the bigger picture" and take a calm view of what really needs to happen. The following steps will help:

★ *Try to find a healthier approach to life's many challenges, so that they do not interfere in the same negative way with your health.*
★ *Keep visualizing your desired outcome and make a note of the steps required to achieve this.*
★ *Break tasks down into manageable, bite-sized chunks.*
★ *Delegate some tasks, if possible.*
★ *Set aside time to constantly review whether the steps you are taking are leading you forward.*

★ *Try to keep emotions running smoothly, looking out for danger signs, such as disturbances in your sleep patterns, food cravings, or even twinges of a headache. These are signs that you may once again be out of balance.*
★ *Remember that you have the internal resources to deal with anything that life throws at you; the secret lies in not allowing your emotions to control you.*
★ *Remain an interested observer of your emotional life, and from this standpoint, your wiser self will know what you need.*

Live in the moment
★ During your daily activities, try to concentrate fully on the task in hand – regardless of how important, or not, you consider it. If you are involved with it, then it warrants full attention.
★ Try not to allow your mind to wander, and if it does, then calmly release the vagrant thoughts – like passing clouds – and bring your focus back to the task in hand. You may find you have to do this many times to begin with, as you try to build up the positive new habits of

focused concentration.

★ Remain fully present in every moment and practise being completely mindful and 100 percent aware of everything you do. It seems that much of our time is spent in "remote" – allowing events to unfold or thoughts to churn around without our full presence. How many times when you are driving, for example, do you arrive at the destination with no recollection of actually driving there? Or how often are you unable to remember what you did only a matter of minutes or hours ago?

★ Give everything you are doing a value and place in your life. If you can find no value in it, it may be worth not repeating it again, as it is wasting your precious energy and probably causing you unnecessary stress.

TUNE INTO YOUR SENSES

Concentrate on every task that presents itself, using each of your precious senses to their full. Practising this regularly will begin to awaken the senses that perhaps lie dormant within you; awakening these will encourage you to exercise more power of choice in what you undertake and what you think about, thus maintaining migraine-free health and balance in the mind and body.

Look
Really look at what is happening around you – taking in detail, colour, and textures.

Listen
Listen carefully to what is going on around you – particularly making an effort to give your full attention to anyone speaking. Try to get a sense of what they are really saying from their perspective. If there is no-one else present, then listen to everyday sounds, trying to differentiate one from another.

Touch
Really feel what is happening – touch with your hands if you are involved in a practical task (even if it's as mundane as doing the washing up); feel and appreciate the ground beneath your feet if you're walking or running, and use your mouth to experience every sensation involved in eating. Feel, too, the air as it enters and leaves your lungs, and tune into the beating of your heart.

Smell
Breathe fully and evenly – in through the nose and out the through the mouth – taking note of all aromas.

Taste
Truly savour the flavour of every food and drink you consume, distinguishing each and every taste from the others.

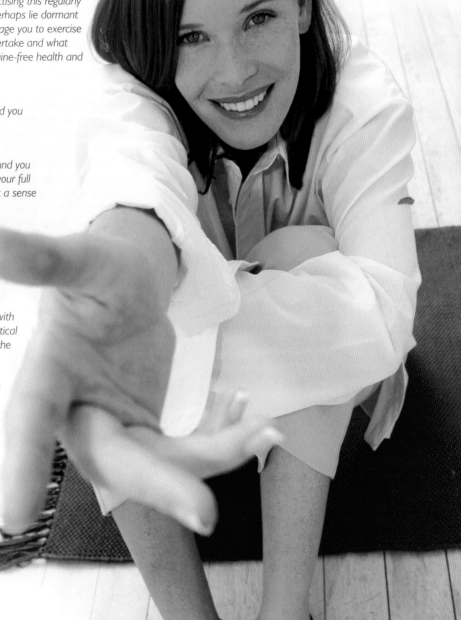

Anger reliever

Anger can build up very quickly at times of stress, causing a build-up of chemicals in the body, which, unless released, can lead to muscular tension, and in turn tension headaches. When such feelings begin to mount, spend a minute or so doing this exercise.

3 *With a strong exhalation, rapidly punch one fist forward, turning the hand over as you do so. Be sure to relax the facial muscles and the jaw as you do this. Draw it back toward your hip again, turning the hand up, on an inhalation. Repeat with the other arm, before doing the whole process several more times. Then do it a few times in a slower, more controlled fashion. Take a few deep breaths to finish and enjoy the feelings of release, as you will have vented pent-up anger with the rapid punching movement and restored a sense of balance with the slower action.*

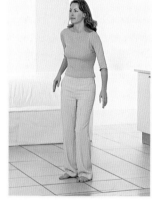

1 *Stand, hip-width apart, and give your body a gentle shake-out to relax and get the blood flowing.*

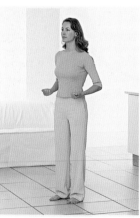

2 *Inhale. Clench your fists, palms up, and draw them back toward your hips.*

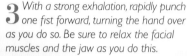

Anger release

It is believed in Chinese healing philosophy that the liver is the organ most likely to suffer from feelings of anger (see also box on p. 14). This links in well to the "liverish" feelings of nausea and vomiting often experienced with a migraine attack.

The following meditation exercise, which is of Chinese origin, is designed to help discharge anger from the liver and to bring about a state of balance, from which healing can arise. It can be done sitting or standing, but if you decide to sit, it needs to be on a chair without arms so that you can move freely.

★ Stand or sit in a relaxed but upright position.

★ Visualize the colour green – the fresh, new green of springtime – as the liver is associated with the wood element, the nature of which is this colour.

★ Take your attention down to your liver – the area immediately below the rib cage, on the right side of your body (see below left) – and flood it with green energy. Aim to breathe into this area, feeling it relaxing, but at the same time energizing it and making its work easier.

★ Raise your right arm in the air and lean to the left, away from the liver, breathing out the sound "shhhh". Concentrate on the liver and absorb this sound into your body, as it has been found to have a natural resonance with the liver, producing a soothing, healing vibration, encouraging it to clear and renew itself.

★ Breathe in as you return to the upright position. Repeat nine times. With each outward breath, release old feelings of anger, and with each inward breath replace them with feelings of gentleness and calm control by breathing in the colour green.

★ At the end of the exercise, spend a few moments in contemplation, feeling the vibrations of the healing sound "shhhh" echoing through your being, chasing away old anger.

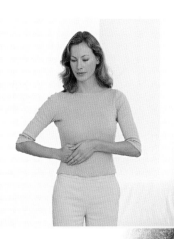

Anxiety reliever

Fear and anxiety can arise from, or create, an imbalance in the energetic flow of the kidneys. Many underlying fears, however, have little foundation in reality, yet lead to tension headaches. The following exercise will help release such habitual fears.

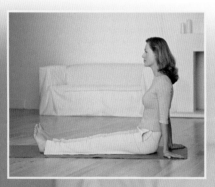

1 Sit on the floor with your legs outstretched, your back upright but relaxed, and your hands on the floor by your hips.
   Visualize a beautiful dark blue – the calm colour of a midnight sky or a still lake. Then concentrate around the area of your kidneys – the lower back – and imagine this area flooding with this blue as you breathe in.

2 Exhale with the sound "whooo" – gently, as though blowing out a candle – while stretching your hands down your legs toward your feet.

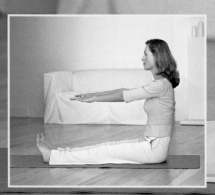

3 Inhale, as you sit upright, still concentrating on the colour blue. Repeat nine times, allowing your fears to release with each exhalation and breathing in new energy with each inhalation.
   Now spend a few moments in contemplation, feeling the vibrations of the healing sound "whooo" echoing through your being, chasing away old fears.

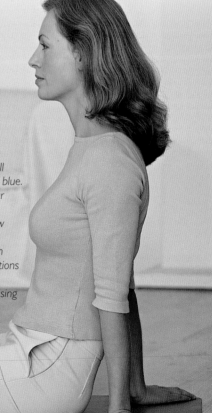

Letting go *of* *grief*

This exercise will encourage a strong flow of energy toward the lungs, which will, in turn, bring about feelings of courage and resourcefulness, helping to dispel the sadness and despair that often accompanies regular migraine attacks.

4 *Spend a few moments in contemplation, feeling the vibrations of the healing sound "sssss" echoing through your being, chasing away old sadness.*

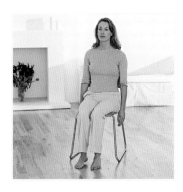

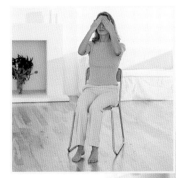

1 *Sit upright in a chair, with your feet on the floor, hip-width apart, your back supported and your arms free to move. Visualize white – bringing cleansing and clarity. Then concentrate on your lung area.*

2 *As you inhale, visualize white light filling your lungs. At the same time, lift your arms up in a wide arc, until your hands are resting lightly on your forehead, palms inward and fingertips gently touching.*

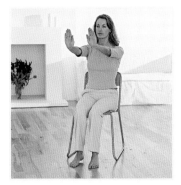

3 *Exhale, with the sound "sssss", while turning to look up, and extending your arms to push your palms away from you.*
Inhale white as you return your hands to your forehead, looking forward again. Repeat nine times in total, exhaling with the sounds "sssss" each time. Allow all sadness to flow out as you breathe out, and encourage strength to flow into you as you breathe in white light.

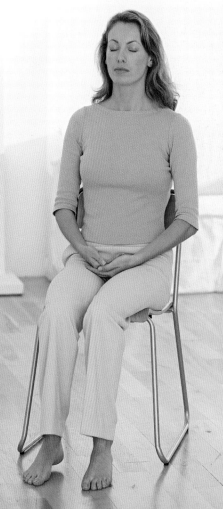

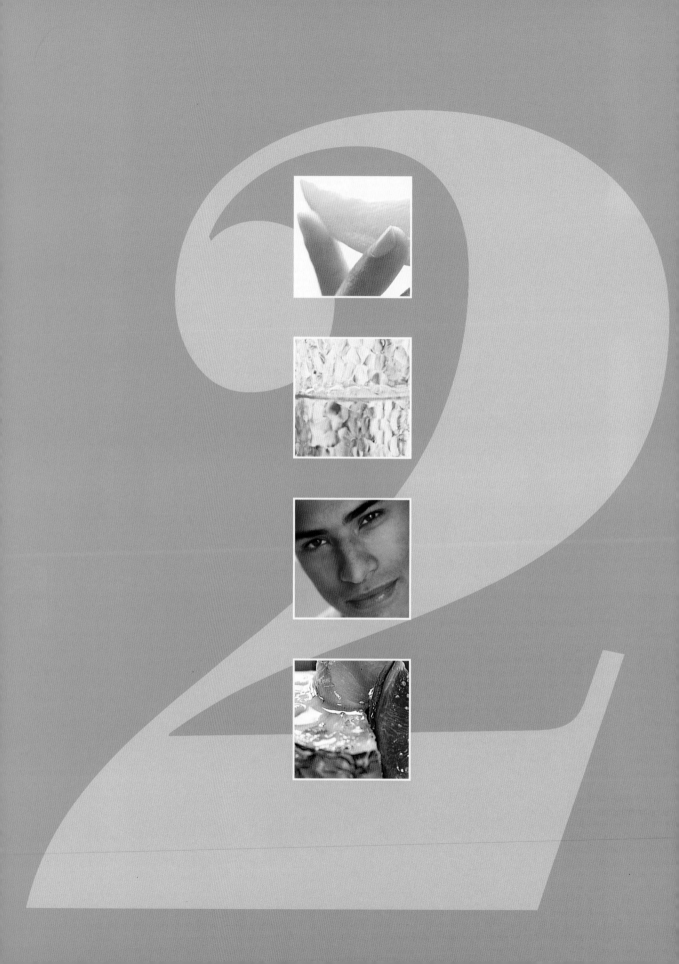

Chapter Two

Looking at your
DIET

---

*It is said that the way
to enlightenment lies in having
a full heart, a full stomach,
and an empty mind*

The importance of diet

Advice about diet and nutrition seems to come at us from so many directions that many people just "switch off" when it comes to yet more "shoulds" and "shouldn'ts", but it's crucial to consider these factors when trying to prevent migraines.

The aim here is not to bombard you with further dietary "do's" and "don'ts", but simply to draw your attention to an awareness that headaches, and particularly migraines, can be an indication that the body is being put under stress by certain foods and drinks – the pain being a signal to stop consuming them. Some migraines can therefore be thought of almost as an "allergic" reaction to certain products; the key is finding what it is you're allergic to and doing something about it.

Healthy eating is not about becoming a slave to dietary rules, but is about developing an awareness of what your body needs – or doesn't need – at any given time. Our mind so often tells us what to eat out of a sense of habit that we may have lost the ability to listen to our body's true messages. These come in numerous forms, including aches and pains, a lack of energy, anxiety, the inability to sleep and relax, and, of course, migraines. The secret lies in learning to pick up on and respond to these signals and to credit your body with the intelligence that it undoubtedly has.

The food factor

The foods and drinks that we introduce into our bodies all have an effect on our quality and flow of energy, or chi (see pp. 9–10). The consumption of healthy food and drinks have a positive effect on our chi, which, in turn, has a positive effect on our overall health.

Conversely, it is believed that the consumption of excess amounts of "unhealthy" foods have a negative effect on the body's energy flow, thus giving rise to ill health, including migraines. Highly processed foods, and artificially stimulating beverages and snacks, such as tea, coffee, biscuits and chocolate, for example, put the body's vital organs and major processes – the heart, liver, kidneys, and digestive system – under great strain. In fact, many of these "unnatural" foods

"Trigger" Foods

Certain food and drinks have been found to be the most common causes of migraine. These include:

* ★ *Coffee*
* ★ *Chocolate*
* ★ *Cheese*
* ★ *Alcohol*
* ★ *Citrus fruits – particularly oranges*
* ★ *Food containing monosodium glutamate (MSG) – an additive that is often used as an appetite and taste stimulant in snacks and fast foods*

actually require more life force to process and eliminate them than they actually supply to the body. As a result of this hard work, the body becomes depleted of chi, causing a loss of vitality and a sense of being "under the weather" in some way, such as in the form of migraines.

Spotting "unfriendly" foods

Let's start with the simple things. It will be helpful if you are able to recognize any foods or drinks that may be acting as obvious "triggers" to your migraine attacks. Look out, during an attack, for any food or drink to which you develop an aversion, in particular something you may have consumed just beforehand and are now unable to stop thinking about. If, however, nothing comes to mind, then it's a good idea to try keeping a diary of everything you eat for a while, looking back at it every time you experience a migraine, to see how your attack fits in with your eating patterns. Alternatively, you may wish to give your body a spring clean (see pp. 26–27), or you may wish to try the food tests on pages 32–35 to try to pinpoint culprits.

Certain foods and drinks are notorious for sparking off migraines (see box left). And unfair though it may seem, these "trigger" foods are often the very foods that you crave or give yourself as a reward.

The list of trigger foods here is by no means exhaustive. We are all complex individuals, with individual responses, so what may be good for one person may be highly inappropriate for another.

Of course, diet is just one of the possible factors behind the onset of migraines, but paying attention to healthy eating will give your general health a boost anyway, so is well worth doing.

FEELING FRUITY

Although it's best to avoid oranges if you're a frequent migraine sufferer, other fruits are very good for you.

Spring cleaning

A very good way of sorting out what food and drinks may be adversely affecting you is to give your body a good "spring clean". This detoxifies your body, allowing you to start with a clean slate and identify anything that causes problems as you reintroduce it.

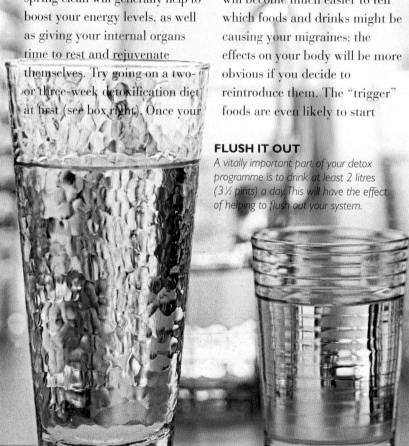

Giving your body a thorough spring clean will generally help to boost your energy levels, as well as giving your internal organs time to rest and rejuvenate themselves. Try going on a two- or three-week detoxification diet at first (see box right). Once your body is clear and balanced, it will become much easier to tell which foods and drinks might be causing your migraines; the effects on your body will be more obvious if you decide to reintroduce them. The "trigger" foods are even likely to start

FLUSH IT OUT

A vitally important part of your detox programme is to drink at least 2 litres (3 ½ pints) a day. This will have the effect of helping to flush out your system.

losing their appeal. For example, your mind may tell you how much you would love to eat that huge bar of chocolate, but you will find that eating it makes you feel ill or sluggish, and this way of feeling will become a guide for you not to have it the next time. To begin with, however, it is strongly advisable to refrain from any of the "trigger" foods while seeking to alleviate your headaches and migraines. You should only resume them, now and again, once you truly feel that your body has had a rest and has been brought back into balance.

Stage 1: Battle through

For a few days at the beginning of your spring clean, you may feel pretty dreadful. Don't worry. This is a good sign: a sign that your body is struggling to rid itself of the toxins accumulated via your habitual way of eating. Your body may start craving foods and drinks that it had developed an addiction to. You may have headaches, be a little nauseous, and feel generally low. The more toxins your body has to rid itself of, the stronger its reactions will be. If it is too dramatic – for example, if you had been accustomed to drinking ten cups of coffee a day and cutting it out completely makes you feel punch drunk – then cut down gradually over several days. Listen to the needs of your body and gently coax it into new, healthier habits. This is likely to create a more effective long-term change; forcing your body to adapt to a new regime too quickly will only cause further stress, and could result in you reverting to unhealthy habits quite rapidly.

Stage 2: Getting there

After a few days of following the eating plan, you will start to feel the benefits, including an overall increase in energy and, all being well, less frequent, less severe, or maybe even no, migraines. Drinking plenty of fresh water will help to speed up the process as it will help to keep flushing the toxins out of your body.

Stage 3: Worth it

After a detox period of two or three weeks you will most likely feel that this process is well worth carrying on with, as you should notice positive changes to the way you feel. Your levels of energy will probably be noticeably higher and the quality of your sleep should be improved. You

---

Detoxing the Body

Below is a summary of the steps you could take – either temporarily or permanently – to give your body a spring clean and potentially find the cause of your migraines:

★ Drink plenty of fresh water – at least 2 litres (3½ pints) a day
★ Avoid refined and processed foods and drinks
★ Buy and eat organic foods, where possible, to give your body a rest from pesticides, herbicides, and artificial additives
★ Have a break from dairy products

★ Eat plenty of whole grains and cereals
★ Eat large quantities of fresh fruits and vegetables, but avoid citrus fruits for a while
★ Substitute red meats with lighter meats and fish
★ Avoid processed meat products altogether

---

may notice that you generally feel brighter, clearer in your thinking, and less prone to bouts of depression or anxiety. Your skin may develop a healthy glow, and your eyes will most likely be shining. Some excess weight – the result of taking in foodstuffs that your body had trouble assimilating – might even have melted away! And, of course, you might even be migraine-free. If not, however, you may need to do further investigation into other foodstuffs, as explained in the section on Testing Food Responses on pages 32–35. But cleaning up your diet will be a good foundation to support the other methods in this book, even if your headaches and migraines do not disappear as a result of it.

Having experienced a sense of well-being from this "spring clean" and having gained, too, a familiarity with how different foods and drinks affect you personally, it may be that you would now be happy to continue

with your new healthy eating programme, assimilating it into your way of life. Alternatively, you may prefer to revert to some of your old eating habits (if they have not lost their appeal) and just have the occasional spring clean when you start to feel sluggish, headachy, or under par. The choice is yours, but what is important is that you develop the awareness that gives you the choice over what you consume, and that you are prepared to really listen in to your body and its constantly changing needs.

It is sometimes the case that straight after a spring clean, when the body has eliminated its residue of toxins, it will happily tolerate just about anything. However, any suspect foods should only be introduced one by one over an extended period of time (if at all), in case you experience an adverse reaction once again.

Making food *work for* you

We are all familiar with the saying "you are what you eat". In view of this we should make every effort to take steps to eliminate as much processed and refined food as possible and replace it with "natural" food – food rich in vital nutrients that the body can easily use to stave off migraines. Ideally, food should be as near to its natural state as possible.

Stay hydrated

Simply drinking about 2 litres (3 ½ pints) of water a day can dramatically improve your health and energy levels – so much so that you will honestly wonder why you didn't try this before. Water is one of the fundamental healers, along with oxygen and exercise, all of which are readily available, and very inexpensive, if only we would embrace them. The benefits are enormous in terms of keeping the vital organs hydrated, in particular the brain, which is the first organ to suffer if the body is lacking in water and which can lead to throbbing headaches. The elimination of toxins is also a lot easier and more efficient when the body is well hydrated, leading to an improvement in the condition of skin and hair, as well as improved concentration. We lose our ability to feel thirst so easily that the body is often in a real state of dehydration before we actually realize that we are, in fact, thirsty. Sometimes the body will even give out hunger signals to attract attention when all it really wants is fluid.

If remembering to drink sufficient water is a problem for you, then try filling a large container every morning as a reminder. Then decant some into smaller bottles to carry around with you during the day – if you take small, frequent drinks while out, you will feel a lot less tired. You will begin to notice that the more water you give your body, the more it wants. Your sense of becoming thirsty will return to you again, as your body begins to work more efficiently.

Plenty of fruit & veg

Lots of fresh fruit and vegetables not only provide a real treat for the body in terms of vital nutrients, but are also a ready source of antioxidants, which combat the inflammation that so often causes migraines. Fruit and veg are good daytime snacks as well as mealtime ingredients – raw carrots, celery, or an apple are particularly good alternatives when you feel the urge for a

WATER FOR LIFE
Drinking plenty of water daily can make a dramatic difference to your well-being and help set the healing process in motion.

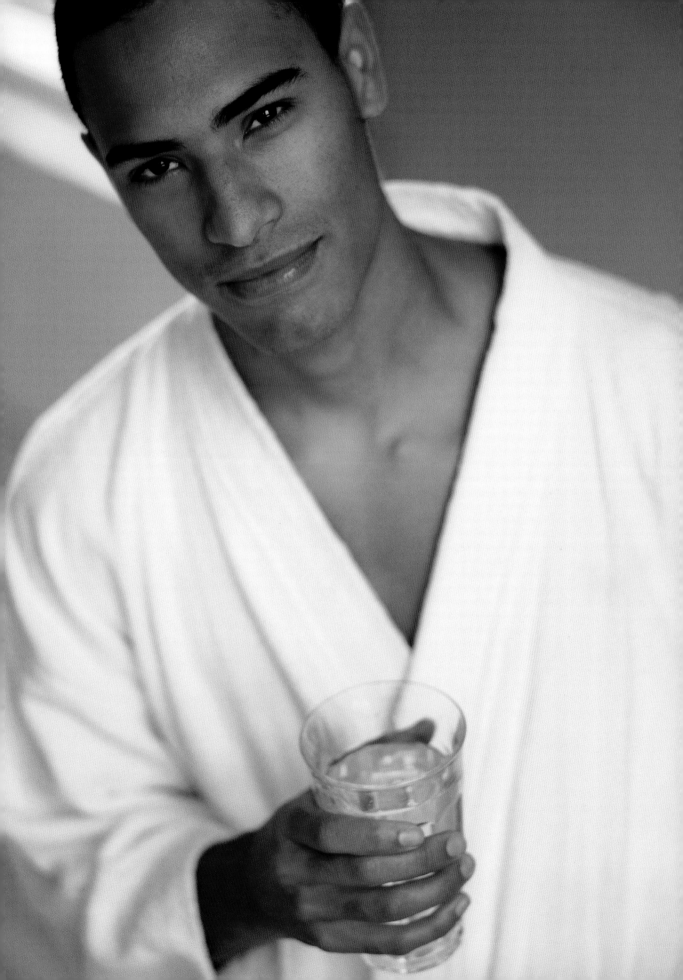

sneaky chocolate bar.

Vegetables are also good for you if lightly steamed or made into delicious soups and salads. Make a habit of having a salad with every meal and fresh fruit at breakfast time. Be adventurous with your salads, as most veg can be eaten raw. Add avocados, nuts, seeds, and chopped fresh or dried fruit, and make them as colourful and appealing as you can. One example would be to chop and grate a selection of root vegetables, and sprinkle them with freshly chopped herbs, olive oil, and black pepper. Delicious!

Feed your body regularly with calcium- and magnesium-rich green vegetables. These minerals are definitely the headache-sufferer's choice, as they help in the prevention of painful spasms. Try making a nourishing drink by juicing spinach, celery, kale, and broccoli, adding lemon juice

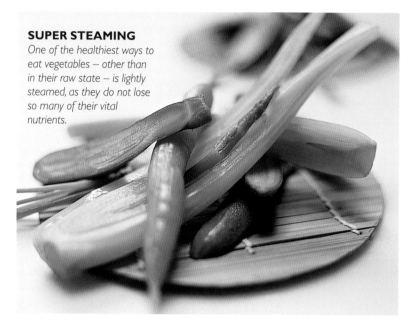

SUPER STEAMING
One of the healthiest ways to eat vegetables – other than in their raw state – is lightly steamed, as they do not lose so many of their vital nutrients.

to taste. This drink will have a soothing, quietening effect on the nervous system, and should be sipped slowly.

Herbal teas, vegetable juices, and fresh fruit juices – with the exception of those made from citrus fruit – can be drunk freely. For further advice and recommendations on the most helpful herbs to take, please look at pages 36–57.

Wholesome health

Substitute refined, white grains with organic whole grains, where possible, and choose brown rice, wholewheat pastas, and brown breads (rather than white). Not only are these much more nourishing – providing a good supply of vitamins, minerals, and proteins, and helping the body to eliminate unwanted toxins – but the body will take longer to digest them due to the

fibre content, so that hunger will be kept at bay for longer. Rushes of energy, followed by slumps, will become a thing of the past, and a more constant flow of energy will take its place.

Pulses and nuts are also recommended. Literally bursting with the vital nutrients we need for good health, they provide a particularly good source of protein, which is especially important for vegetarians.

Anti-inflammatories

Foods with anti-inflammatory properties can be extremely beneficial to migraine-sufferers, as headaches are often caused by inflammation. Fresh ginger and garlic are useful for this reason: try a stir-fry of freshly chopped seasonal vegetables, lavishly flavoured with fresh garlic, root ginger, and a handful of cashew nuts. Essential fatty acids found in seeds, nuts, and oily fish are

Importance of Regularity

Ideally, eat three regular nourishing meals a day with wholesome snacks in between, if you get hungry, such as fruit, nuts, or raw veg. This will help to keep the blood sugar levels constant. You will find that if your eating is irregular or high in sugar and refined carbohydrates, your blood sugar levels will fluctuate dramatically, causing distress to your body and increasing the likelihood of migraines. Try never to allow yourself to get too hungry. Carry some emergency food rations around with you if necessary.

Diet Summary

The lists of foods and drinks below are reminders of the foods that it's best either to steer clear of or eat a lot of when trying to beat debilitating migraines:

Avoid:

★ Refined or processed foods
★ White sugar
★ Potential "trigger" foods, such as tea, coffee, chocolate, cheese, oranges, fizzy drinks, and alcohol
★ Dairy products
★ Wheat products, if there is a sensitivity toward them
★ Red meat
★ Foods from the nightshade family, such as aubergines, tomatoes, peppers, and potatoes
★ Sweets, chocolate, biscuits, and cake

Embrace:

★ Fresh and dried fruit
★ Fresh vegetables – especially ones that are rich in calcium and magnesium, such as broccoli, kale, and spinach
★ Whole grains
★ Seeds and nuts
★ Fish, especially oily fish; flax seed oil for vegetarians
★ Lean, white meat
★ Soya products
★ Occasional eggs
★ Honey instead of sugar
★ Herbal teas and lots of fresh water

also useful anti-inflammatories. Also try avoiding, for a while, foods from the nightshade family such as tomatoes, potatoes, aubergines, and peppers. These can all contribute to an inflammatory state in the body.

Dairy don'ts

An occasional break from dairy products can be very beneficial for the digestive system. These foods produce a lot of mucus during digestion and can also produce an inflammatory reaction, which can lead to headaches and a "sluggish" feeling. Some migraine-sufferers are allergic to cheese and cream, but are able to tolerate low-fat milk products, or even goat's or sheep's milk. Otherwise, try substituting dairy products with

soya products every now and again. Experiment by using tahini or houmous as a substitute for butter and trying soya ice cream or yogurt as an occasional treat. Coconut milk or soya

yogurt is delicious with fruit salad or with muesli (and fruit) for breakfast.

Keep it light

Replace rich, heavy red meats with fish and poultry – organic where possible. The body takes a long time to digest red meat, causing a sluggish feeling. This "heaviness", and any resulting illnesses, can be avoided by sticking to lighter alternatives.

Ideal substitutes

Use honey as a sweetener instead of sugar, which is a stimulant, causing unnecessary strain on the vital organs. Drink fresh fruit and vegetable juices, herbal teas, and plenty of water instead of tea, coffee, and fizzy drinks – often key migraine "triggers". Avoid alcohol, as it causes strain on the liver and may cause headaches.

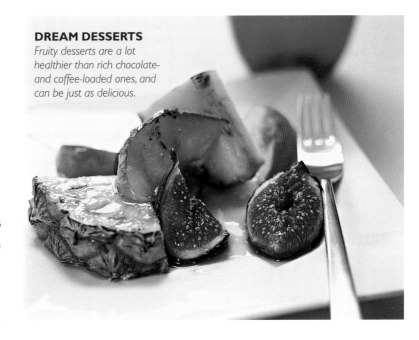

DREAM DESSERTS
Fruity desserts are a lot healthier than rich chocolate- and coffee-loaded ones, and can be just as delicious.

Testing food responses

It is possible to test your natural response to the foods and drinks you consume by testing your body's instinctive reaction to their presence. The exercises on the following pages – the "Strong Arm" test and the "Finger Pull" test – will allow you to do this simply.

If we consume something that our body is unable to tolerate, it causes a weakening significant enough to be revealed by the following tests, which are used by many health practitioners.

The "energy tests", or chi tests, can be a very useful personal guide and may be thought of as a tool for translating the energy messages of the body into a simple physical indication of what is good for you and what is not. Learning to "energy-test" your foods will give you a different relationship with the foods you eat. Very often, you will start to lose interest in foods that cause a depletion in your energy levels and/or imbalances in your body that lead to pain – migraine or otherwise.

Having said that, a healthy body will be able to cope with a certain amount of junk food.

Becoming too obsessive about what you can or can't eat is in itself a stress, and the idea is to free ourselves up from too many inappropriate stresses. The aim of the following tests is therefore simply to find out whether the energy – or energetic vibration – of certain foods is in harmony with our own energy, or vibration. If it is in harmony, it will be good for you, and if it isn't, it will be bad for you – it's as simple as that! This can be a

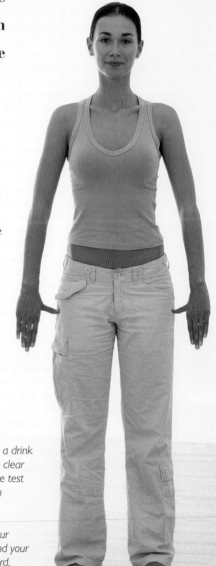

THE STRONG ARM TEST

Do this test with a partner and have a drink of water beforehand. You should both clear your minds of any expectations of the test results as the mind can interfere with the body's real messages.

1 *Place your hands by your sides. Your thumbs should touch your legs, and your fingers should point straight downward.*

2 Your partner places their hand between your body and your arm, at wrist height. At a given signal, your partner starts to apply slow, even pressure to try to lift your arm away from your body. Try to resist the movement of your partner, while keeping your elbow straight and your body relaxed. Neither of you should use a lot of strength and you should not struggle to keep your arm in place by recruiting any other muscles. If your arm lifts up rather than staying firmly in position, you should both adjust your resistance levels until it stays in place. This is the "control" test.

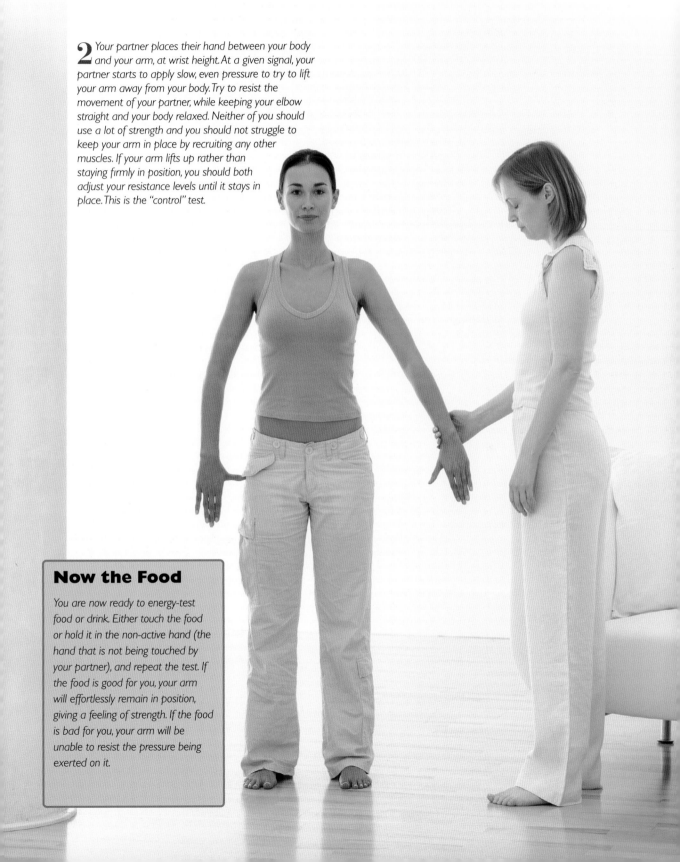

Now the Food

You are now ready to energy-test food or drink. Either touch the food or hold it in the non-active hand (the hand that is not being touched by your partner), and repeat the test. If the food is good for you, your arm will effortlessly remain in position, giving a feeling of strength. If the food is bad for you, your arm will be unable to resist the pressure being exerted on it.

quick and useful way of unearthing all kinds of allergies or intolerances of which you were previously unware, but which had been draining your natural forces and causing migraines. You will find that your body's needs and reactions vary with time, affected by numerous factors such as stress levels, quality of sleep, fitness levels, and external factors such as pollution and your environment. There are likely to be certain foods to which you always react badly and which you should therefore always avoid. However, there are others from which you probably only need a rest, and which you may be able to assimilate again at some time in the future, if you want to. It is therefore worth trying the tests with the same foods at regular intervals – perhaps weekly or monthly, or when you feel your body has had a bit of a rest from the foods with which it was initially having problems.

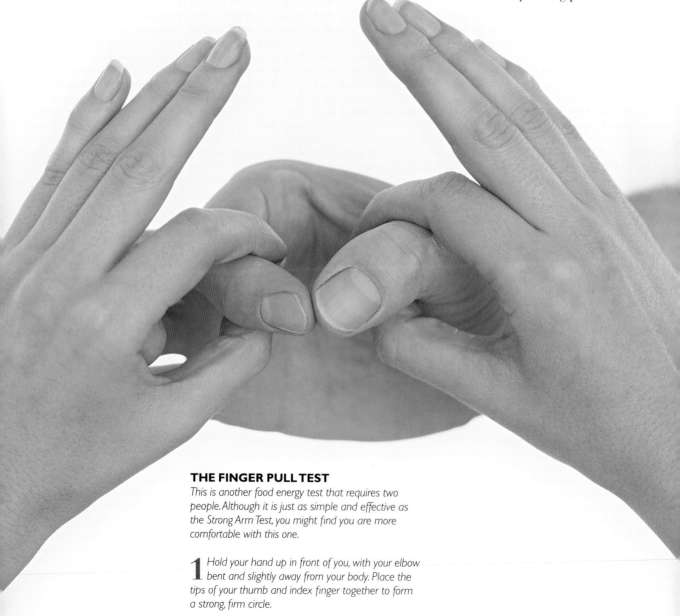

THE FINGER PULL TEST

This is another food energy test that requires two people. Although it is just as simple and effective as the Strong Arm Test, you might find you are more comfortable with this one.

1 *Hold your hand up in front of you, with your elbow bent and slightly away from your body. Place the tips of your thumb and index finger together to form a strong, firm circle.*

Top Tips

★ *Drinks can be tested the same way by simply either dipping a finger in it beforehand, or by placing a few drops on the hand.*

★ *These energy tests can also be used for testing the suitability of supplements, remedies, and anything else that you may be uncertain about taking or consuming.*

★ *The presence of metal will nullify these energy tests, as it has a particular effect on the body's energy. So move away from metal kitchen implements and kitchen foil, remove any metal jewellery or accessories that you are wearing, and make sure you remove the food you are testing from any metallic packaging.*

2 *Your partner should use his index fingers and thumbs to create two circles linked though your circle. He should then try to break your circle with these, without jerking or using unreasonable strength. If the circle breaks easily, you are not using enough resistance or your partner is using too much force. This should be adjusted accordingly before doing the same test again with a piece of food in your free hand.*

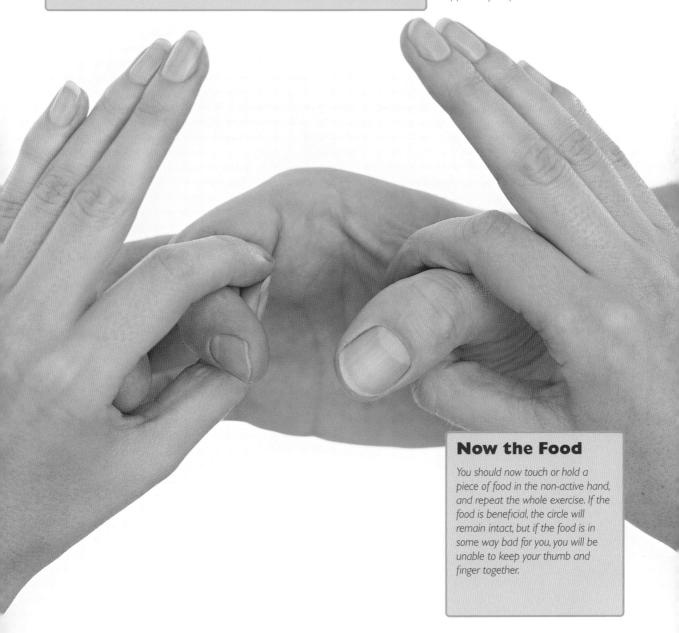

Now the Food

You should now touch or hold a piece of food in the non-active hand, and repeat the whole exercise. If the food is beneficial, the circle will remain intact, but if the food is in some way bad for you, you will be unable to keep your thumb and finger together.

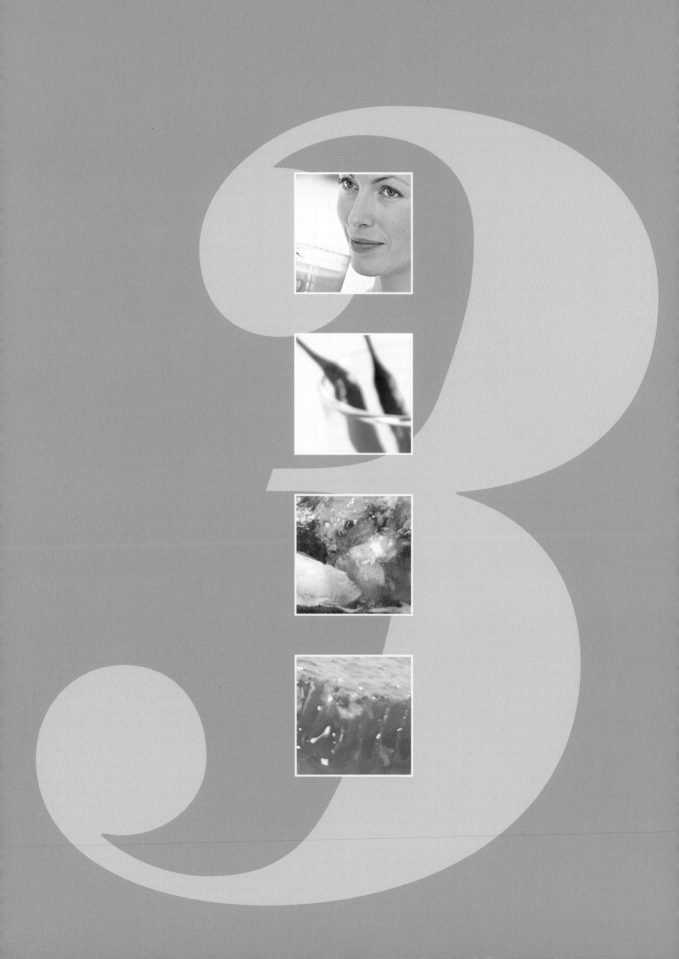

Chapter Three

JUICING

your way to health

Bursting and brimming with
freshness and fruitiness,
deliciously smooth,
pure zest for life

Delicious smoothies
juices &

Believe it or not, investing in a juicer or blender could be a really beneficial long-term health move. This is because fruit and vegetables are so good for us (see pp. 28–31), and raw fruit and vegetables are even better. Cooking destroys many of their vital elements, while whizzing them up in the blender lets us keep these "goodies", helping us stay healthier.

Raw fruit and vegetables in juice form is simply great for you. You can often feel the benefits of a vitamin- and mineral-packed juice almost instantly – you are nourishing your body with so many nutrients that it can't help but benefit from an increase in energy almost straight away.

The liquid form means that myriad nutrients can be delivered almost immediately into the bloodstream, giving the body minimal processing to do. Juices also allow you to take in larger quantities of fruit and veg than you could if you were to sit and try to plough your way through platefuls of actual food.

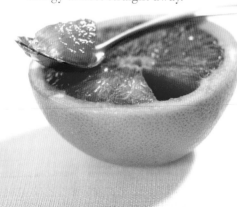

RAW GOODNESS
Juicing allows the fresh nutrients of raw fruit and vegetables to get into your system quickly and directly.

Mixing it up

You can experiment and make up your own juice recipes from the list of useful ingredients (see pp. 40–41) or you can follow the specific recipes on the following pages. Foods that are naturally rich in calcium and magnesium are particularly helpful for headache- and migraine-sufferers, as they have been found to reduce distressing and uncomfortable spasms. These minerals can be found in many fresh fruits and vegetables.

Making up a fruit smoothie as a breakfast substitute is a nourishing way to greet the day: it will be so packed with fresh nutrients that it should happily keep your body ticking over for a while. If you are avoiding dairy products, however, try substituting standard milk with soya milk, rice milk, or oat milk. Soya milk is particularly beneficial in the case of hormone-related headaches; rice milk is a great source of B vitamins and

Top Tips

★ *If a vegetable juice seems too strong a flavour at first, use pure spring water to dilute it.*

★ *Use honey to sweeten and lemon juice to sharpen.*

★ *Drink the juices immediately if possible, as keeping them for more than about 15 minutes significantly reduces their nutritional value. Unfortunately, these fresh juices do not keep well refrigerated, so cannot really be prepared in advance. However, they are so quick and easy to make, and so delicious, that it really isn't a chore to just whizz them up!*

fresher, and your headache may well be a distant memory.

Prep

Buy organic foods for juicing when you can and wash all ingredients thoroughly in hot water before using. This washing stage is particularly important if you are unable to buy organic products. Alternatively, try the following method of getting rid of surplus chemical deposits – add two tablespoons of salt and the juice of two lemons to a pot of cold water and soak your fruit and vegetables in the mixture for ten minutes, before rinsing them with cold water, ready to use. The quantities suggested in the following recipes are sufficient for up to two glasses, but can be

minerals, and oat milk is soothing for the nerves in the case of a stress-related headache. Alternatively, add the slightly more exotic almond milk for a really delicious treat.

It could be good to make up a fruit smoothie for breakfast and a vegetable juice for later on in the day. For a quick afternoon or evening pick-me-up, try juicing three or four carrots – perhaps adding half an apple to taste. This works wonders for a toxic type of headache – perhaps one brought on by an over-indulgence in rich food or alcohol – as it is a wonderful cleanser. Within five to ten minutes of drinking it, you should feel brighter,

varied to suit the individual.

Remember that every person is different and will therefore have different reactions to the juices – in terms of both preferred flavours and therapeutic effect. You might find one or two that work particularly well for you and stick to those, or you may even find that it is best if you adapt one of the recipes slightly to suit your needs. Become adventurous at inventing your own recipes. Use the following list of suggested ingredients to inspire you and see how many varied and interesting tastes you can come up with.

Best fruit & veg
Fruit and vegetables rich in calcium and magnesium are great in juices for migraine-sufferers: cauliflower, celery, broccoli, spinach, corn, apples, bananas, kelp (seaweed), sunflower seeds, sesame seeds, and brown rice (as in rice milk).

Hot tips
"Hot herbs" such as ginger, cayenne, and hot peppers or chillies are surprisingly effective for relieving congestion headaches, particularly following a cold or flu. They should be used with caution, particularly if used in powder form, as they can be very hot.

Other "goodies"
★ *All fruits and vegetables* are good, apart from any you may be trying to avoid for a while, such as oranges. Bananas are a particularly good source of potassium.

★ *Dried fruits* are an excellent

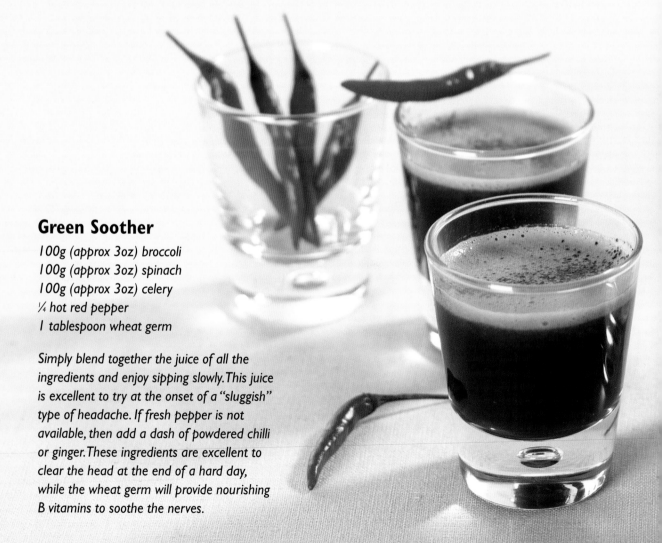

Green Soother

100g (approx 3oz) broccoli
100g (approx 3oz) spinach
100g (approx 3oz) celery
¼ hot red pepper
1 tablespoon wheat germ

Simply blend together the juice of all the ingredients and enjoy sipping slowly. This juice is excellent to try at the onset of a "sluggish" type of headache. If fresh pepper is not available, then add a dash of powdered chilli or ginger. These ingredients are excellent to clear the head at the end of a hard day, while the wheat germ will provide nourishing B vitamins to soothe the nerves.

source of vitamins and minerals, plus their natural sweetness provides a boost to blood sugar levels. Soak in fruit juice for a few hours before use.

★ *Wheat germ* is rich in B vitamins and is especially good in the case of "nervous" headaches.

★ *Oat milk* is a rich source of B vitamins.

★ *Soya milk* is helpful for menopausal and pre-menopausal headaches if drunk regularly. Try to buy soya milk that has been fortified with calcium, for added benefit.

★ *Almond milk* is a delicious and valuable source of protein.

★ *Avocado* is an effective source of protein and is very rich in a variety of vitamins and minerals – particularly potassium, which is essential for a healthy and balanced nervous system.

★ *Iron-rich foods* such as brewer's yeast, dried apricots, kidney beans, parsley, and dark, green-leafed vegetables such as spinach and watercress are all valuable ingredients to juice when you have a low-energy headache or one resulting from long-term fatigue.

★ *Aloe vera*, renowned for its anti-inflammatory properties when used as an external ointment, is now available as a juice and is a very good "tonic", particularly for convalescence. This is because it contains such a wide range of nutrients – B vitamins, vitamin C, and many minerals such as calcium, magnesium, and iron. Try drinking on its own, as prescribed on the container, or adding it to vegetable juices for a real boost to the system.

Sweet Smoothie

1 banana
200 ml (⅓pt) soya milk
1 tablespoon sunflower seeds
1 teaspoon honey

This sweet, calming juice is really easy to make – simply whizz up the ingredients in your juicer and you're set. Just make sure you use soya milk rather than "real" milk as dairy foods have been known to trigger migraine attacks. The proportions of the ingredients can be varied according to taste, and you can feel free to add a couple of strawberries or raspberries for extra sweetness and luxury if you like, as well as for a splash of colour. The calcium- and magnesium-packed sunflower seeds can be added at the end if you prefer a crunchier texture.

Fatigue-fighting juices

When you think your migraines may result from stress and general fatigue – the sort of exhaustion that just isn't helped by a few good nights' sleep – try making juices from ingredients rich in iron, calcium, magnesium, zinc, and essential vitamins.

Examples of these foods are seeds and nuts, apples, bananas, peaches, avocado, carrots, celery, spinach, broccoli, cabbage, watercress, beetroot, oats, brown rice, soya products, algae, and parsley. Try a glass of a juice made from one of these at the end of a tiring day – it will help stave off fatigue and lift your headache, particularly if you relax and sip your juice slowly to savour the benefits. Alternatively, try the following energizing recipes.

Veg Delight

100g (approx 3oz) carrots
60g (approx 2oz) cabbage
60g (approx 2oz) beetroot
30g (approx 1oz) watercress
30g (approx 1oz) parsley
1 teaspoon sesame seeds

A wonderfully fresh-tasting, green pick-me-up, this is bursting with energizing nutrients and is perfect for fatigue-related headaches and low energy. Juice the veggies and blend all the ingredients together.

Fruit Fantastic

1 banana
1 apple
1 peach
1 tablespoon mixed nuts or seeds
200 ml (⅓ pt) soya or rice milk

This smoothie tastes of pure luxury – a real treat either at breakfast or at the end of the day. It is bursting with calcium and magnesium, both really helpful to treat tight headaches with pains that come and go, and the nuts and seeds provide added protein. Juice the apple and peach and blend with the other ingredients.

Stress-busting *juices*

For headaches and migraines resulting from feelings of stress, tension, and anxiety, you need something that will calm your nerves and relieve the effects of the excess adrenaline in your system. Fresh juice is a perfect way to deliver this almost instant nutrition.

A lack of minerals in the diet, such as iron, calcium, and magnesium, can lead to an increase in stress symptoms, so replacing the missing nutrients can be a good way to get on the road to recovery. There are many foods that can help do this, from algae, ginseng, brewer's yeast, and aloe vera, to seeds, nuts, brown rice, wheat germ, dried fruits, soya products, oats, broccoli, bananas, apples, spinach, beetroot, parsley, and watercress.

Go Green

100g (approx 3oz) celery
60g (approx 2oz) spinach
30g (approx 1oz) watercress
1 teaspoon parsley
1 teaspoon alfalfa

This drink is packed full of iron and calcium to help soothe exhausted or shattered nerves. Stress is a major contributor to headaches and migraines, and this juice will help to thoroughly nourish the nervous system, alleviating stress. Add black pepper to taste. Juice and blend all ingredients.

Apple & Apricot Alleviator

120g (approx 4oz) soya, oat, or rice milk
6 dried apricots
1 apple
1 tablespoon brewer's yeast

Pre-soak the apricots in a little apple juice – perhaps overnight – before juicing and blending the ingredients together. You can either use commercial apple juice for this soaking stage or you can make your own by juicing a couple of apples. Brewer's yeast and both rice milk and oat milk are full of nerve-soothing B vitamins and make a delicious drink when blended with fruit. This recipe suggests apricots for the iron content and apple for the vitamin and calcium content, but you could use other fruits if you prefer. Try, for example, using dried figs – previously soaked in apple juice – with banana. This is heaven – guaranteed to soothe stress-related headaches.

Hormone-balancing *juices*

Fluctuating hormones may be an underlying cause of some migraines. This can be helped by including an abundance of fresh foods in your diet. Avoid too much fat, eat plenty of fruit and vegetables, and include both soya products and foods high in fibre.

Whole grains and soya products are good in hormone-balancing juices in your juice mixes, as are foods rich in calcium and magnesium, such as wheat germ, nuts and seeds, leafy green vegetables, and sea vegetables, such as spirulina, kelp, and dried seaweed. Also use ingredients that act as natural diuretics in order to reduce the discomfort of pre-menstrual swelling. Particularly good ones for this purpose are grapes, watermelon, cucumber, celery, parsley, and watercress.

Try drinking pure watermelon juice or grape juice, but not too much as they are high in sugar and can lead to further bloating if taken in excess. Leave in the seeds when you juice these fruits, because, like other seeds, they are a good source of minerals. Alternatively, try the following recipes:

Green Goddess

120g (approx 4oz) celery
100g (approx 3oz) kale or spinach
60g (approx 2oz) alfalfa sprouts
1 small teaspoon of spirulina or kelp powder
Lemon juice to taste

This is an excellent combination to help prevent irritable, period-related headaches and to help combat cravings often accompanying pre-menstrual symptoms. Spirulina and kelp are rich sources of trace minerals, including iron, which is particularly valuable for menstruating women. Celery, kale, and spinach are rich in calcium, and alfalfa sprouts, when available, provide a ready source of protein.
Juice the celery, kale, and sprouts before blending with the other ingredients.

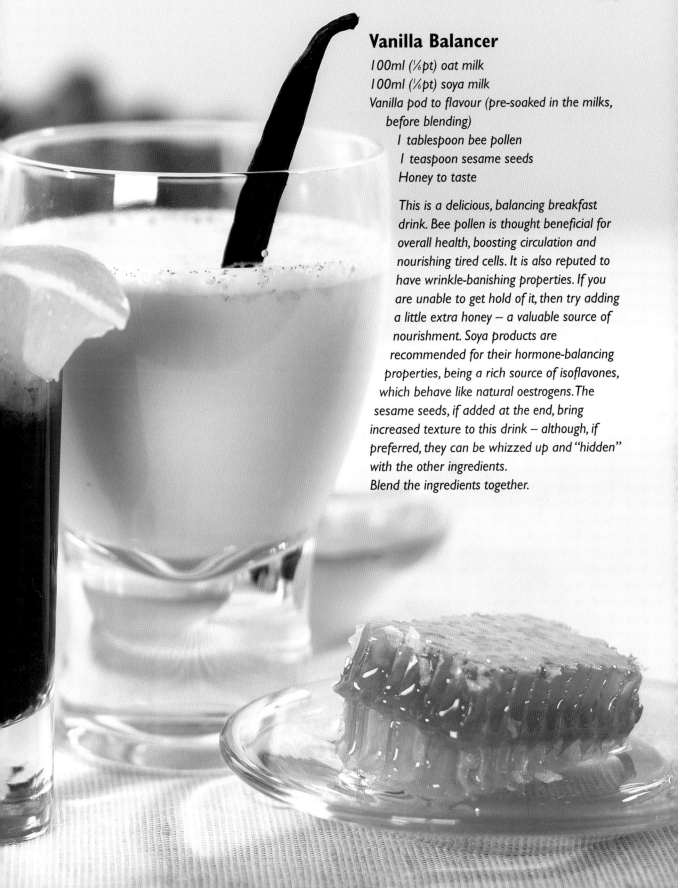

Vanilla Balancer

100ml (⅙pt) oat milk
100ml (⅙pt) soya milk
Vanilla pod to flavour (pre-soaked in the milks,
    before blending)
    1 tablespoon bee pollen
    1 teaspoon sesame seeds
    Honey to taste

This is a delicious, balancing breakfast
drink. Bee pollen is thought beneficial for
overall health, boosting circulation and
nourishing tired cells. It is also reputed to
have wrinkle-banishing properties. If you
are unable to get hold of it, then try adding
a little extra honey – a valuable source of
nourishment. Soya products are
recommended for their hormone-balancing
properties, being a rich source of isoflavones,
which behave like natural oestrogens. The
sesame seeds, if added at the end, bring
increased texture to this drink – although, if
preferred, they can be whizzed up and "hidden"
with the other ingredients.
Blend the ingredients together.

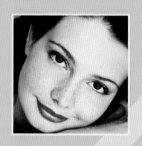

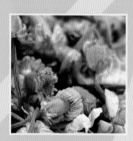

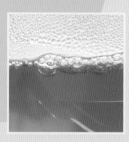

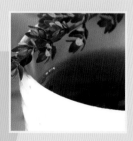

Chapter Four

Making HERBAL REMEDIES

In Mother Nature's lore,

opening the doorway

to her boundless gifts of healing

Herbal *brews*

The use of herbs and plants for their therapeutic qualities is an ancient art, which has enjoyed a revival in modern times. Much valuable knowledge has been handed down to us through the years, and a lot of this ancient wisdom has now been scientifically researched and acknowledged. It is very much accepted that certain plants can have a measurable effect on our health, and, indeed, many of them now form the basis of modern-day medicines.

Herbs can also be used to great effect in more traditional ways, such as brewing them into teas (see pp. 52–57) or adding them to the bath for a relaxing soak. Although there are still specialist suppliers of dried herbs, many are now quite readily available in health food stores. Try hunting in garden centres for some of the more unusual varieties. Alternatively, you may even like to grow them yourself, either in the garden or in containers – perhaps outside the kitchen door or on the window sill. This way you will have a ready supply of herbs, which you could dry by tying bunches together and hanging upside down in a warm, dry spot. When they are dried, store them in airtight containers and use as required.

Herbal bath

The quiet warmth of a bath will help to soothe away aches and pains, but adding a therapeutic brew of herbs to your bathwater will bring even more pleasure. The aromas can do much to lift the spirits and ease away painful headaches. All you need are some fresh or dried herbs and some hot water – as simple as making a cup of tea, except that you use a stronger mix than for tea and you steep it in the boiling water for longer.

Add the ripped leaves or dried herbs to a pot of water, cover, and simmer on a low heat for several minutes. Leave to steep for twenty minutes off the heat, strain, and add to a warm bath. Then relax into the water and breathe deeply, inhaling the healing properties of the herbs.

★ Ginger is wonderful, but should be used with caution as it can sting a little if it is too strong. It helps dilate the blood vessels and can therefore help prevent migraines. It is also effective for headaches that are the result of exposure to the cold or congestion of the sinuses and is also good for general invigoration, leaving you tingling all over. Try taking a ginger bath two or three times a week, but not while you are actually suffering from a migraine attack, as it would be too stimulating and may produce feelings of nausea.

Grate or finely chop about 5cm (2in) of fresh ginger and simmer for about twenty minutes in a litre (1¾pt) of water. Strain and add to a warm bath. Then relax in the water for at least ten minutes.

★ A mixture of **chamomile, lavender, and marjoram** is great for a relaxing bedtime bath. It will gently ease stress and tension out of weary muscles, relieving headaches, and calming the nervous system. Use about a handful of fresh herbs or a couple of tablespoons of dried herbs, to about half a litre (1pt) of boiling water. Try this bath two or three times a week as a preventative measure against migraine – but only between attacks. It can also be useful at the onset of a headache

as it will help to relax the body, and the gentle aromas will help to still a racing mind.

★ **Rosemary,** renowned for its mildly stimulating properties, is good for a pick-me-up bath when your headaches leave you feeling a bit low or "sluggish". Add approximately two tablespoons of the dried herb or a good handful of the fresh herb to half a litre (¾pt)of boiling water. Try at the onset of a headache caused by too much mental activity, which may have left you feeling fatigued and muddle-headed.

★ A mixture of **rosemary, ginger, and peppermint** is wonderful for headaches linked to tired, aching back muscles. Use about 2 ½ cm (1in) of fresh ginger, grated or chopped, and gently simmered in water for approximately 20 minutes. Meanwhile, take about a tablespoon and a half of dried herbs or a handful of fresh herbs and steep them in boiling water. Strain both mixtures and add them to your bath – pure bliss.

ENJOY A HOT SOAK
There is nothing more relaxing than a deep, luxurious bath – particularly at the end of a long hard day, when your limbs are aching and your head is throbbing.

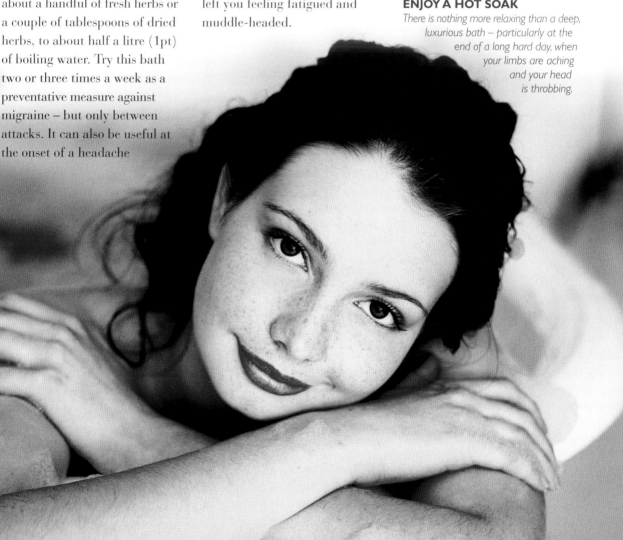

Herbal teas

Herbal teas are a simple and pleasant way of introducing therapeutic herbs and plants into our regular diet. There are many herbs that can be useful to help prevent, or at least alleviate, the pain and discomfort that comes with migraines, and there are other herbs that are better for their more long-term preventative properties. Some herbs, however, should not be taken during a migraine attack, as they may be too strong and cause feelings of nausea.

It is wonderful to drink a brew of freshly picked leaves, but dried herbs can be just as effective if fresh herbs aren't available, depending on the season and your proximity to health stores and garden centres. However, most of the more common herbs can now even be bought as tea bags. This is certainly the case for peppermint, rosemary, chamomile, and feverfew, all of which are helpful in the case of migraines and headaches, and are quick and easy to use.

The therapeutic properties of the most useful herbs to prevent or relieve migraines are explained in the following pages, along with a few effective anti-migraine recipes to try. You should soon find the ones that work best for you – and of course that you enjoy most. But feel free to experiment a little with the ingredients suggested to cater fully for your own needs.

What to do

To make a herbal tea, simply place a spoonful of dried herb, or a small handful of the leaves of fresh herbs, into a container; add hot water and leave to stand, covered, for three to four minutes. It is important to allow the herbs to infuse in the water for this time, rather than boiling or simmering them, as they are often fairly volatile and much of their therapeutic value could be lost in this way. You can vary

Which Herbal Tea When?

Most herbs are therapeutic, whenever you decide to take them. However, some can be too strong to take during a migraine, so use the information below as a guide.

Migraine prevention:	Onset of migraine:	During migraine attack:
Feverfew	Passiflora	Chamomile
Thyme	Chamomile	Peppermint
Basil	Lemon balm	Rosemary
Dandelion root		Vervain
Marjoram		Passiflora
Vervain		

the amount of herbs to alter the strength of the tea, according to taste, and honey can be added to sweeten.

Rosemary

Rosemary is a powerfully aromatic herb, which is excellent for bringing relief from congestion headaches, caused by prolonged mental activity. It is a great cleanser, having antibacterial properties, and its powerfully woody, herbaceous aroma helps to lift the spirits, encouraging renewed concentration and stimulation of the mind. Rosemary should be avoided during pregnancy, as well as by people with epilepsy, due to its strong properties.

Vervain

Vervain is an important herb for use in the relief of headaches and migraine – particularly stress – and nerve-related ones – due to its ability to relax the muscles, calm the nervous system, and help promote sleep. This herb is also a good digestive tonic, due to its bitter properties, and is therefore also helpful in the prevention of headaches and migraines caused by poor or sluggish digestion.

Feverfew

A very important herb to try, feverfew is extremely beneficial in the alleviation of migraine as it has been found to directly improve the blood circulation to the brain. It should be taken in a tea two or three times a day – rather than once migraines have already set in – as it is particularly helpful as a preventative measure. However, the effects take a while to become apparent – so be patient.

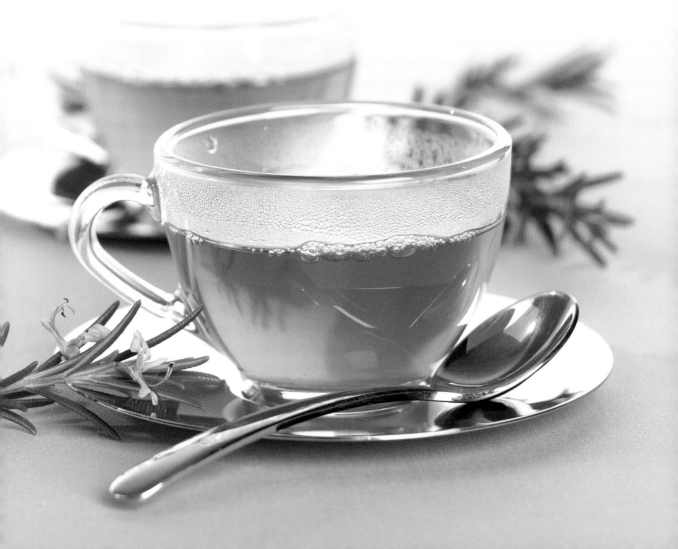

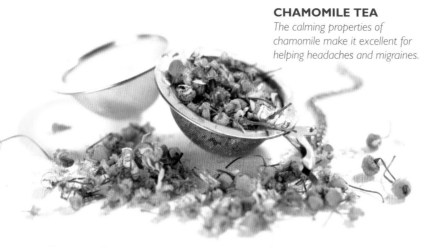

CHAMOMILE TEA
The calming properties of chamomile make it excellent for helping headaches and migraines.

Dandelion

Dandelion root is a well-known tonic for the liver, helping to disperse toxins. It is readily available as a pleasant-tasting drink – dandelion coffee. This root is an excellent remedy for digestive disturbances and is particularly useful as a preventative treatment for migraines caused by sluggish digestion and an over-toxic system.

Passiflora

Renowned to be one of the most relaxing herbs for the nervous system, passiflora is often used to promote sleep. It is gently soothing to an over-anxious or worried mind, readily bringing about a state of calm. Passiflora is of particular value in the prevention and treatment of headaches and migraines brought about by tension and stress. It should, however, be avoided during pregnancy.

Chamomile

This is one of the most widely used herbal teas because of its many healing properties. It is gently soothing to the nervous system, helpful in promoting sleep and relaxation, and eases away tension and irritability. Chamomile is particularly helpful in treating headaches that are the result of over-excitability. Its pleasant taste and aroma also make it suitable for children, particularly if sweetened with honey.

Lemonbalm

This delicious-smelling herb will do much to relieve the pain and discomfort of a migraine attack or headache. It has a pleasant, lemony taste, which helps to settle digestive upsets, is one of the easiest herbs to grow, and produces a gorgeous scent in the garden. A handful of dried leaves is also a great way to keep your wardrobe smelling fresh.

Peppermint

One of the most well known herbs is peppermint, which is refreshing, very effective, and will help to settle the stomach in the case of "tummyish" headaches, where nausea and possibly even vomiting may accompany the pain. Peppermint is useful for helping to break down fatty or oily foods in the digestive process, thereby helping the liver to work more efficiently. The refreshing properties of this herb help to bring about a feeling of alertness and vigour, while its minty fragrance lifts the spirits, banishing any feelings of sadness and depression.

Ginger

Ginger crops up regularly in the pages of this book – and with good reason. It has wide-ranging digestive benefits and is excellent for problems relating to poor circulation, as it promotes bloodflow to the extremities. This makes it a very valuable remedy, both internally, in the form of tea, and externally, in the form of herbal baths and compresses.

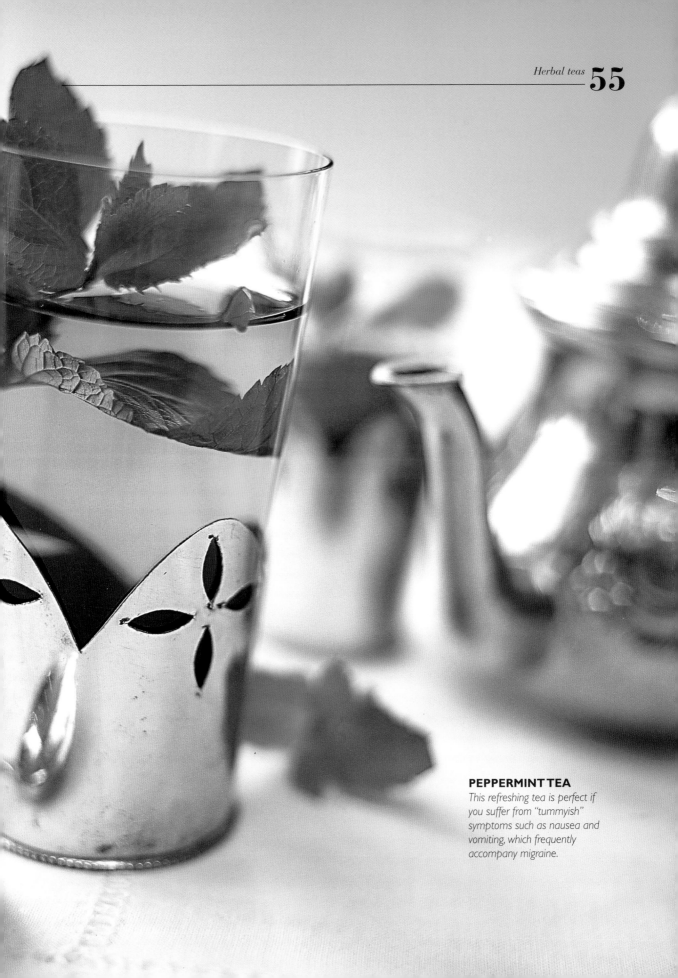

PEPPERMINT TEA
This refreshing tea is perfect if you suffer from "tummyish" symptoms such as nausea and vomiting, which frequently accompany migraine.

Migraine-busting infusions

Nature can provide us with a range of effective remedies to help soothe debilitating chronic conditions such as migraine. It is well worth trying the following herbal infusions as a preventative measure between migraine attacks.

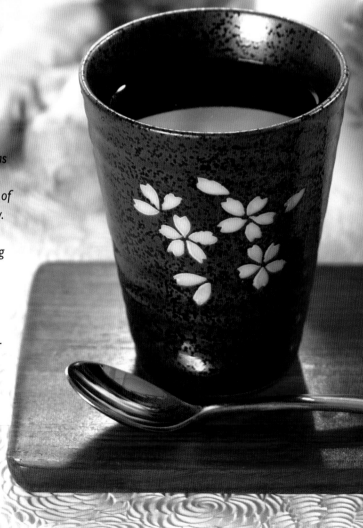

Pain Wizard

The combination of ingredients in this infusion makes it aid the digestive process as well as soothe away unnecessary tension. This makes it especially helpful in the relief of migraines brought about by nervous anxiety.

It is best to take this mixture every morning when you get up and every evening before retiring to bed over a period of two weeks. Enjoy!

Take half a flat teaspoon of each of the following herbs: vervain, chamomile, thyme, and basil. Infuse them in a cup of hot water for five minutes. Strain, and drink immediately. Again, this tea can be sweetened with honey, if desired.

Chinese Magic

The Chinese have long been renowned for their skills and knowledge in herbal lore. The following is a recipe of Chinese herbs, which can be used to great effect for a "liverish" migraine attack, helping to detoxify the liver, thereby assisting efficient digestion and bringing the body into balance.

Its benefits are gradual so you should drink it several times a day over a period of weeks or months before you really feel the effect. Most of the ingredients should be available at local health stores, but otherwise, seek out specialist herb suppliers, especially Chinese herbalists.

Take a teaspoon of each of the following herbs: verlain, dandelion root, ginger root, marshmallow root, motherwort, and centaury. Add them to a pot containing about one litre (1 ¾ pt) of water, cover, and simmer for about 15 minutes on a low heat. Strain, and drink one cup before each meal. Keep the remainder refrigerated, and heat as required. It can be sweetened with honey to improve the flavour.

Ginger compress

Compresses are a traditional method of treating painful conditions, and are made by applying a hot or cold cloth to an area of distress. Adding therapeutic herbs to the infusion into which we dip the cloth makes compresses all the more effective.

Ginger has long been viewed as a valuable therapeutic herb by Chinese medical practitioners. Records of it go back some three thousand years and its effects are far-reaching. As seen on page 51, it can be used to great effect as a herbal addition to a soothing bath. However, it can also be used externally in the form of a compress on the skin due to its heating and restorative properties. It is particularly useful in the treatment of strain due to the cold or tightening of the muscles. This is because it creates warmth in the area, increasing the blood flow, easing congestion, and relaxing muscle spasm. It can also be useful as a comforting and therapeutic aid to detoxification if placed over the liver – the area just below the rib cage, on the right side of the body. You should experience a pleasant heat and tingling sensation for quite a while after using a compress. And all of these therapeutic effects will help to combat your migraines. Place it over the liver area every morning and evening for two weeks. If you think, however, that your pain may be stemming from a stiff or painful neck or shoulders, it is better to use it across the neck or on the shoulders instead – either at the onset of a headache or as a preventative measure.

Making the compress

It is really very quick and easy to make an immensely soothing ginger compress.
★ Add a dessertspoon of dried ginger or a 5–1-cm (3- to 4-in) piece of fresh ginger, grated, to a pan of water.

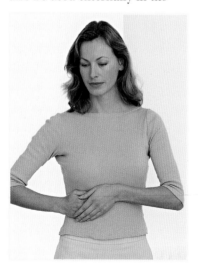

THE LIVER AREA
Locate your liver area on your lower right side, just below your ribcage.

Cover the pan and simmer the mixture slowly for 20 minutes to extract the therapeutic properties.

Then allow it to cool enough to remain hot, but not scalding.

★ Next, dip a cloth into the brew – a piece of towelling is ideal because it is dense enough to hold the heat.

★ Wring the cloth out thoroughly and apply it either across the neck and shoulders for muscle-related headaches or on the area of the liver for migraines that feel as though they are more related to internal body processes. The compress should feel hot to the touch, but not to the point of feeling uncomfortable or burning the skin.

As the cloth cools down, soak it thoroughly in the ginger water again. Keep repeating this until the water is too cool to be effective – most likely after about five minutes.

The ginger water can be kept refrigerated and reused several times, heating it each time until it is hot to the touch.

SOOTHING COMPRESS
Use a soft towel or flannel for your compress as this fabric will hold the heat for longer. As it cools, repeatedly dip it into the brew so that you get maximum benefit from it.

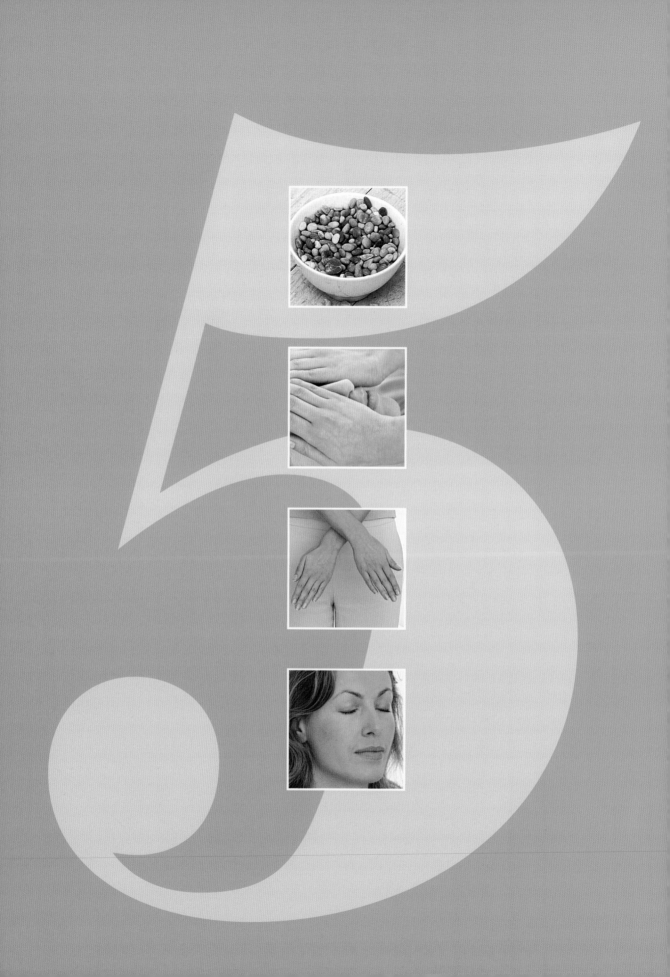

Chapter Five

RELAXING
your way
to health

In the quiet of your innermost being

know that all is well,

from the depths of your soul

feel at one with all that is

Winding *down*

Most of us are all too familiar with the adverse effects of stress – modern life often seems to conspire to "wind us up". So for many of us, developing the ability to cope with stress will play a large part in helping prevent headaches and migraine attacks.

It is unrealistic to try to remove stress completely from our lives, because we find that it is often the very factor we need to encourage us to make changes and to develop. Stress, in itself, can be a great motivator, as it causes chemical changes to arise in the body that support action and activity. Problems only arise when you "sit on" these chemical changes, for whatever reason, not making the decisions that

you need to in order to utilize the surges of energy. They can then backfire, producing feelings of negative stress and leading to conditions of "distress", with symptoms that include physical illness – in particular headaches and migraines, but also lethargy, depression, outbursts of anger, and a general inability to cope.

This chapter suggests specific techniques to combat the negative effects of stress and the

feeling of being "wound up" by life. However, if you have been following some of the other suggestions in this book, the chances are that you are already becoming more "wound down" as many of them are designed to release feelings of stress and tension in one way or another.

Coping strategies

When life feels like it's all getting too much for you – whether at work, at home, or elsewhere – it's a good idea to break things down into more manageable, bite-sized chunks, reminding yourself that nothing is too much to cope with and prioritizing what you really need to do.

Forget about what may or may not happen next week, next year, or in ten years from now. That is, in the future. Equally, forget about what happened yesterday, last month, or five years ago. That is in the past. All that is really important is what is happening here and now, in this moment. This, you can cope with. If you can get the here and now right, the future is

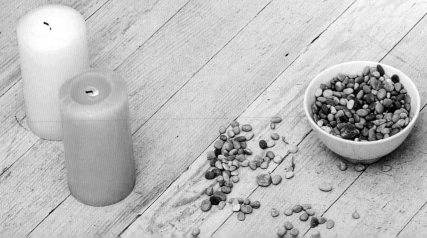

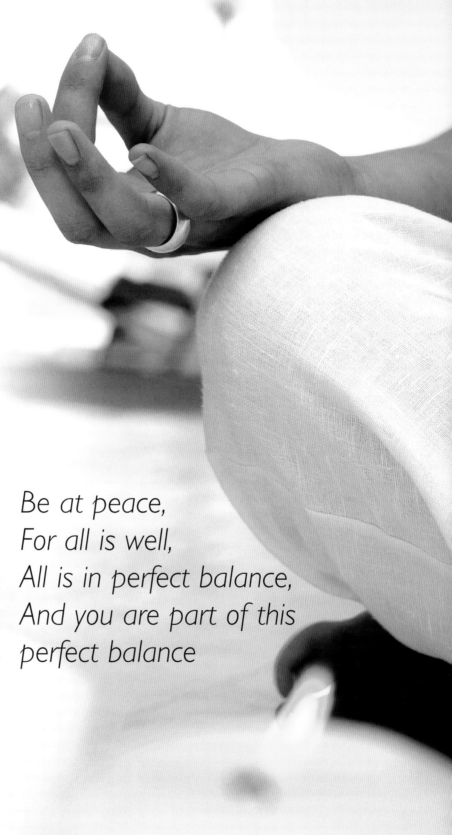

much more likely to work out more or less how you want it to.

Take time to organize your thoughts into what are real problems and what are merely imagined or perceived ones, and waste none of your time and energy on the latter.

Learn to play, learn to relax, and learn the art of contemplation and meditation. This will encourage personal transformation by giving you the choice over whether you participate in the mad, headlong dash of life, or whether you periodically choose to step away from it. Learning to become habitually more relaxed gives you the underlying energy to be much more focused and effective at the times when you need to be.

Perhaps you feel that you do not have the time or inclination to relax and meditate. The time you spend, however, will be repaid to you many times over in terms of clarity of thought, improved sleep, increased energy levels, an improved sense of well-being, and a lack of migraines – all being well! It is therefore well worth the effort to make some time for yourself – even if it's only ten minutes or half an hour a day. Allow yourself this time to truly switch off from all of life's pressures, to still the mind, and to simply relax and exist in the purity of the moment. The exercise on the following page is one for you to try during such a period.

Be at peace,
For all is well,
All is in perfect balance,
And you are part of this
perfect balance

The *dragon breathes into the* earth

Allow yourself half an hour of quiet, uninterrupted time to do the following relaxation technique. Remember that the body loses heat during relaxation, so make sure that you will be warm enough while lying down.

The exercise is simple. All you need to do is lie on the floor or on a mat, allow your body to relax, and then breathe in and out evenly and gently from the abdomen. You will be guided as to where you should direct your breath and provided with visualization techniques to help increase your sense of complete relaxation and tranquillity. Try to remain fully aware of the weight of your body at the various stages throughout the relaxation process: heavy at first, but each area of the body becoming lighter as you focus your breath through it.

2 *Imagine you are able to breathe in through the sole of your right foot, drawing your breath up your leg and visualizing pure white light following the breath. As you breathe out, expel old energy, letting it sink deep into the earth for renewal. Repeat several times, until you feel your leg relaxing fully.*
Then repeat several times on the other leg, too. Be aware of your legs feeling light, energized, and relaxing more fully now.

1 *Lie down on the floor. Stretch each of your limbs in turn and allow your body to sink into the ground as it begins to relax. Focus on the awareness that "breath is life".*

3 Now take your attention to the palm of each hand in turn, drawing fresh energy into your arms, and releasing old energy into the earth as you exhale. Be aware of your arms feeling light, and energized as they relax into the floor.

4 Next, take your attention to the crown of your head. With each breath, feel that you are drawing energy down through the crown of your head, flooding your senses and clearing your busy mind. Have the awareness of drawing pure, white light into your torso. Allow the light to release old energy, doubts, fears, and all darkness. Allow it to sink deep into the earth, as you breathe out. Revel in this state of fresh energy and the peace it brings.

5 From your state of complete relax- ation, feel your whole body breathing in energy and light, and continuing to release – deeper and deeper – layers of dark shadows and old energy. Your whole body is inhaling and exhaling, feeling wonderfully cleansed and at peace.

6 Now take your attention down into your abdominal area, the seat of your vital energy, and visualize a ball of white, blue, or gold light: white for cleansing and renewal, blue for healing and protection, or gold for peace and wisdom. As you breathe into it, see it growing gradually bigger. All of a sudden, allow it to burst, flooding your entire being with glorious light. Bathe in this energetic light, take several, full breaths, and become aware of the weight of your body, as it lies on the floor.

7 To finish rub the palms of your hands together and place them over your closed eyes. Draw the warmth from your palms into your eyes and, when you feel ready, open your eyes and blink into the darkness of your hands. Remove your hands in your own time. Then have a good stretch, and luxuriate in the feelings of renewal and well-being. A drink of fresh, cool, water will complete the process.

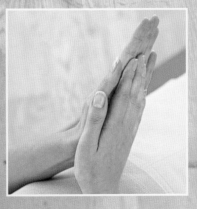

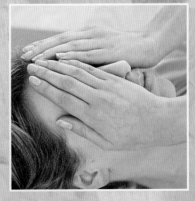

Breath *is* life

Breathing is so fundamental to life that we often take it for granted. But many healing arts, such as yoga and tai chi, stress the importance of correct breathing in relation to our health. And good-quality breathing can help alleviate various conditions by directing chi to specific body areas.

It is frequently the case when suffering with a condition such as a migraine that instinct makes us tense up, as if trying to draw away from the pain. When this happens, the breathing becomes shallow, ironically making the pain worse. Full and relaxed breathing is therefore a simple way to help the body unwind – the best foundation for coping with or seeking relief from pain.

Ways of breathing

Many people do not use the full capacity of their lungs, instead breathing shallowly in the upper part of the chest only – "chest" breathing. This quickly leads to a loss in vitality as we need to take air right down into the lungs – abdominal breathing – in order to get an efficient oxygen supply into the bloodstream. Poorly oxygenated blood causes general sluggishness, contributing to feelings of being under the weather. You will quite simply feel more energized if you breathe deeply. Try the "breathing test" below left to become more aware of this.

Generally speaking, the more tension and stress you carry, the more likely you are to focus on shallow chest breathing. Young children and more relaxed people, on the other hand, tend to breathe more fully, with the focus down in the abdomen.

Just breathe

One of the simplest things we can all do to improve our health, therefore, is to breathe deeply and fully. Learn to enjoy and appreciate the feeling of filling your lungs with air. Know that, with every breath, energy is enter-

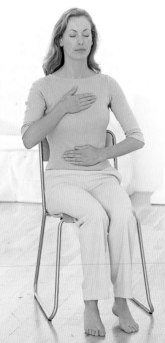

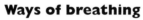

BREATHING TEST

Sit quietly and breathe in your normal way, without attempting to make any judgements or changes. Place one hand over the area of your chest, and the other one lower down, over the abdominal region, and continue breathing. Which hand is moving? Is it the one over your chest, the one over your abdomen, or both? If your upper hand is moving significantly more, you should spend some time trying to breathe more fully and deeply, down into your abdomen (see exercise right).

ing your body and oxygen is entering your blood stream, nourishing your vital organs.

Specialized breathing

There are many specialized ways of breathing designed to help with particular health problems. These techniques work by opening energy pathways through the body – which may have been inactive for some time – thus encouraging a healthy flow of energy to all the major functions and helping to release chronic tensions. The breathing exercises described on the following pages have been drawn from Chinese yoga.

They are simple to do and are very helpful in the treatment and prevention of migraines.

Focus the mind

While practising the exercises, it is important to maintain a state of relaxation, because any tension will immediately prevent vital energy from flowing. The mind, too, plays an important role, as it is also able to direct or "block" energy flow. It is therefore important to focus your mind on the exercises as you go through them – the more you are able to enjoy them, the more benefit they are likely to have.

If the mind wanders off, the

vital energy will follow it. If you are doing a balancing posture in yoga, for example, and allow your mind to wander off – perhaps distracted by a noise, movement, or unexpected thought – focus is lost and you are likely to topple over. This is because concentration and chi leaves the centre and the body follows. It may seem complicated, but if you just relax, breathe fully, and gently keep your mind on what you're doing, you'll be meditating before you know it.

Remember that "breath is life" and that by learning to breathe deeply and fully and practising some exercises, you can very quickly and effectively improve your health and hopefully alleviate, or even prevent, the onset of migraines.

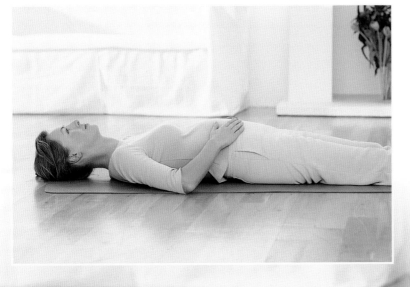

ABDOMINAL BREATHING
Lie on the floor, focus your breathing down into your abdomen, and place both hands gently over this area. As you inhale, feel your belly rise, and as you exhale, feel your abdomen sinking down again. Continue for a few moments, enjoying this gentle movement. This is the type of relaxed, healthy breathing that you should aim to maintain throughout your daily activities.

The joy of life

This is a refreshing, reviving, balancing, and joyful breathing exercise that should be practised every morning and evening, if possible. It is excellent as part of a long-term preventative programme for migraines, and people who do it often feel revitalized afterward.

This exercise gently squeezes and releases the neck and shoulder muscles, and lifts the rib cage, stimulating the digestive processes. It also encourages deep breathing by opening up the chest and lungs. People who suffer from migraines often feel anything but joyful, but this technique will promote a feeling of expansion and happiness in the moment. The emphasis should be on breathing as deeply as you can without strain, and timing the movements with the breath in order to gain the utmost benefit. You may find when you first attempt this that you run out of breath before the movement is finished. This is often because of tension that you are carrying, so the more you relax, the slower and more even your breathing will become.

1 *Stand with your heels together, your toes apart, and your arms down by your sides. Or, if this feels uncomfortable, then just place your feet about hip-width apart. Focus your attention on relaxing.*

2 *As you inhale, cross your right hand over your left in front of you and raise the arms. Allow the cross to deepen toward the elbows.*

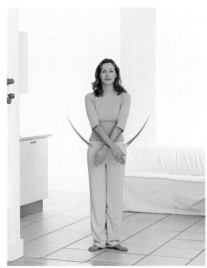

5 *As you gain confidence, stretch up onto your toes when you lift your arms. This will encourage a healthy flow of energy throughout your entire body.*

3 *Then, still on the in-breath, let the arms uncross as they are stretched above your head, palms facing. Your eyes, and therefore your head, should follow the movement of the hands.*

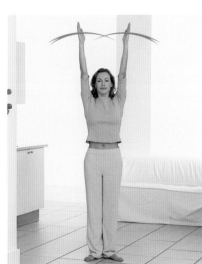

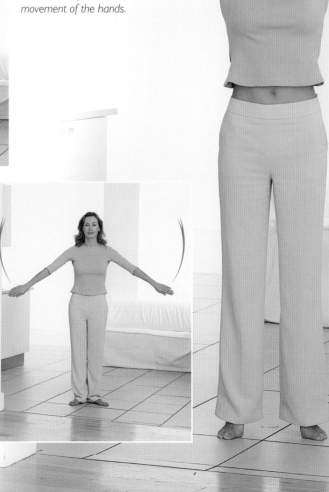

4 *As you exhale, circle your arms down to rest by your sides. Repeat, crossing the other hand in front this time, and, again, timing the large, circular movement to coincide with one inhalation. Exhale as before. The whole process should feel continuous, breathing fully, without strain. Begin with six repetitions, but build up to twelve over time.*

The 4 planes

This is a wonderfully simple exercise to encourage a healthy, harmonious flow of energy around the head, neck, and shoulder region, which is where many people carry a lot of their stress and tension. This tension can build up to chronic levels over time, restricting bloodflow and potentially causing severe headaches and migraines.

It is important to breathe deeply and freely throughout the exercise, as this will allow your natural energy to flow freely into any restricted areas.

The exercise is particularly effective for headaches and migraines arising from muscular tension in the neck and shoulders and from mental overload. Practise the simple movements morning and evening, or at any time during the day when tension is building up. Feel the tension melting away – allow it to simply drip off your shoulders and flow away. This exercise can be either performed standing or sitting upright in a comfortable chair.

A Word of Warning

As with all exercise, be guided by the messages arising from your body. If you have neck problems, other than the normal levels of tension, then proceed with care and caution.

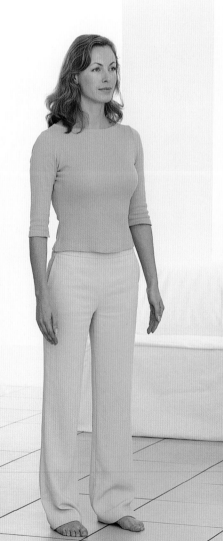

1 *Extend the crown of your head upward, slightly tuck in your chin, and relax your shoulders and arms. Encourage deep breathing by consciously inflating your abdomen with each inhalation and deflating it with each exhalation.*

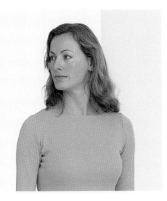

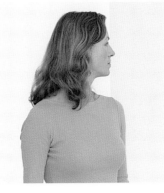

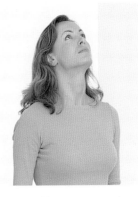

2 *As you exhale, begin to turn your head toward your right shoulder, keeping your neck gently elongated. Be sure to time this movement with the breath.*

Inhale, return your head to the point where you are looking forward again.

3 *Exhale, turn your head toward the opposite shoulder.*

As before, return your head to the centre on the next inhalation. Keep movements gentle and flowing, and time each one with the breath.

4 *Exhale, and keeping your neck extended, tilt your head back slightly, leading with the chin, so that your neck does not become compressed.*

Inhale, return your head to the central position again.

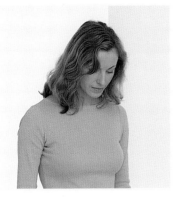

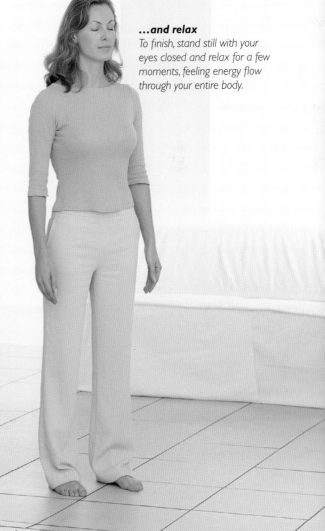

...and relax
To finish, stand still with your eyes closed and relax for a few moments, feeling energy flow through your entire body.

5 *On the next exhalation, take your chin down toward your chest, until you feel a gentle stretch in the back of your neck. It should feel as if it is being drawn down by an invisible thread.*

On the final inhalation, look forward once more. Repeat the sequence three times, building up to six.

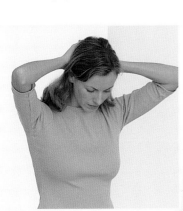

6 *As an extension to this exercise, link your fingers behind your neck at the base of the skull. As you exhale, push your head backward, while pulling the hands forward. Relax as you breathe in, releasing the pressure. Continue several times.*

Encircling the earth

This is one of the most effective breathing exercises for the prevention and relief of migraines and headaches accompanied by nausea and vomiting. It can be practised regularly as a preventative measure, but is also well worth trying at the onset of a migraine, in order to catch it before it develops into a full-blown attack.

Very often, migraines – when not associated with problems in the back, neck, or shoulder region – stem from poor digestive processes, notably of the liver. The exercise on the right stimulates the digestive process and is therefore highly effective in relieving gastric upsets, "butterflies in the stomach", and bowel irregularities. Full and relaxed abdominal breathing (see pp. 66–67) encourages healing energy in the body and therefore forms the foundation for this exercise, as does the use of a pressure point known as the "great eliminator" (see below).

The "great eliminator"

The pressure point known as the "great eliminator" is very useful to become familiar with. As its name suggests, it helps the body to eliminate toxic build-ups and invasion from foreign bodies, such as cold and flu bugs. It is possible to stave off a migraine attack or a headache accompanied by vomiting or nausea by simply relaxing and massaging this point on both hands for a few minutes.

★ To locate this point, place your thumb alongside your index finger. You will notice a slight bulge appearing between the two at the base of the thumb.

★ Now separate your thumb and finger and place the thumb of your other hand in between them to locate a tender point along the index finger edge.

★ Massage gently into the point, using sufficient pressure to produce a mild, but useful, aching sensation. Continue for a few

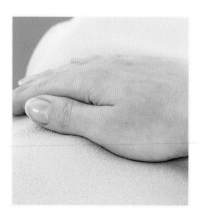
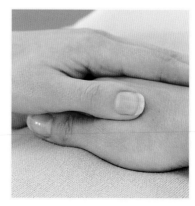

LOCATION
The pressure point known as the "great eliminator" is located on the inner edge of the index finger. Applying pressure here helps eliminate negative energy and therefore associated discomfort.

minutes, breathing deeply and focusing your attention on the sensation being produced.
★ Then locate and massage the pressure point on the other hand.

Simply doing this "great eliminator" massage can bring relief from pain or discomfort quite quickly, but people vary vastly in their responses to such techniques, so it may require a little time before you notice any changes. This simple pressure point massage can also be effective for alleviating other disorders. Try massaging it if you feel under the weather with symptoms such as poor digestion, tummy upsets, sore throats, or even toothache. If, however, this massage is not helping you in any way with your migraines, you may wish to progress to using the "great eliminator" as part of the "Encircling the Earth" exercise below.

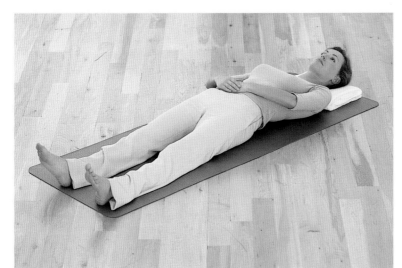

1 Locate the pressure point known as the "great eliminator" (see p. 72) and place both hands against the lower abdomen, with the palms flat down.
  As you inhale and allow your abdomen to inflate, start to massage the area in a clockwise direction – in tune with the natural flow of the digestive tract – moving first up the right side.

2 As you breathe out, continue the massage down your left side, toward the lower abdomen again, making sure that you maintain firm contact with the "great eliminator" throughout.

3 Complete two more circles, timing the movements with the breathing, and applying comfortable pressure. Moving your hands in this circular motion is a symbolic reminder of the Earth element, which is also the element linked to the stomach and digestive process.
  Now change the hands over, enabling you to locate the "great eliminator" on the other hand. Repeat the same circular massage in a clockwise direction another three times, keeping your breathing steady, constant, and in time with the movement of your hands.

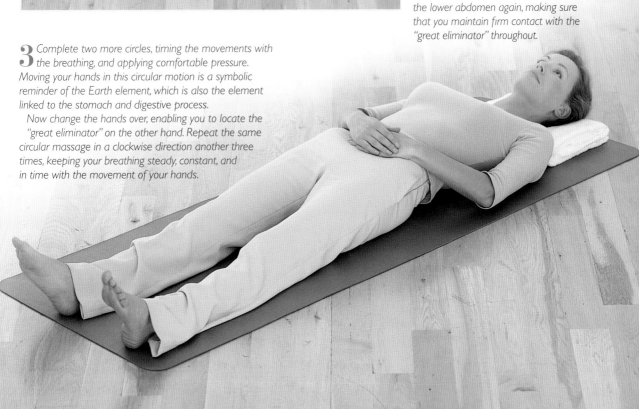

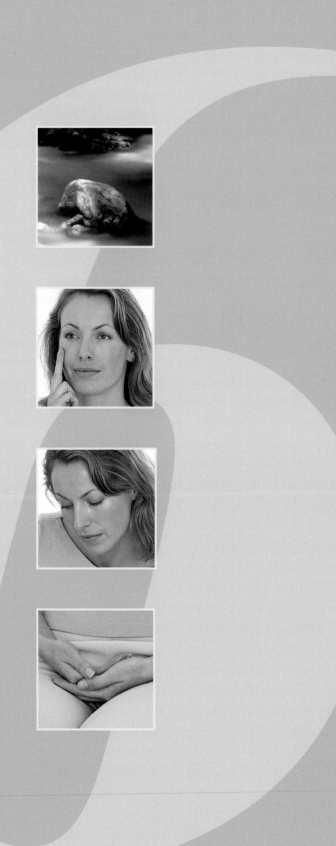

Chapter Six

MASSAGING

your meridians

---

*Tracing paths of energy
and weaving through chaos
to find peace in a healing touch*

Chinese meridian massage

The more relaxed you are, the more evenly and strongly your energy will flow. Tension, on the other hand, produces energetic imbalances and blockages, which often lead to migraines. These can be corrected using simple meridian massage techniques.

It has been claimed by Chinese therapists that migraine attacks can be stopped in their tracks by simply massaging the relevant meridian lines – the twelve recognized energy pathways within the body (see right).

In much the same way that veins and arteries carry blood around the body, meridians are the channels through which our personal energy, or chi, flows, affecting every function of our body. At times, these meridians may become either overactive, underactive, or even blocked, thus not functioning efficiently. If you think of the meridians as a transportation system for chi, it becomes clear that congestion or breakdown can occur, just like in any transportation system. When this happens, the flow of life force to different areas of the body is affected, and illness can result if left uncorrected.

Ebb & flow

Just as the flow and force of a river varies – at times being full and rising, and at other times quiet and shallow – the energy flow in the meridians is also ever changing, affected by myriad influences and conditions. The daily stresses most of us face in our lives, as well as emotional disturbances and physical factors – such as the quality of our diet – are all enough to send our subtle energetic systems haywire. The more we learn to relax in the face of everything life throws at us, and the happier and more accepting we are, the stronger and less susceptible to becoming imbalanced our chi flow will become.

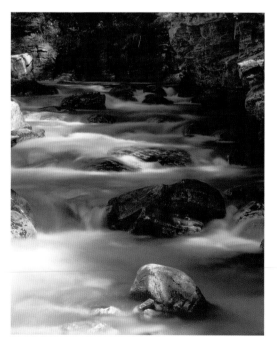

ENERGY FLOW
The flow of energy in the meridians is like the never-ending flow of a river – sometimes fast, sometimes slow.

Pressure points

Although meridians are, in general, not visible, they can in fact be measured by mechanical instruments as they emit electromagnetic energy. Certain points along them can be stimulated with acupuncture needles or by using pressure from the fingers in order to redistribute or redirect the flow of chi.

Self-massage along these pathways (see pp. 78–81) is a very good way of getting things flowing harmoniously once again and will greatly help in the prevention and alleviation of migraine attacks. It is a very simple procedure and need only take a few minutes.

These meridian flushes should ideally be carried out as a preventative measure twice daily for two weeks, once daily for another two weeks, and every other day for a further two weeks. By the end of this period, you should notice a lessening in the frequency and severity of your migraines. But if you feel the need, continue to incorporate the massages into your daily routine.

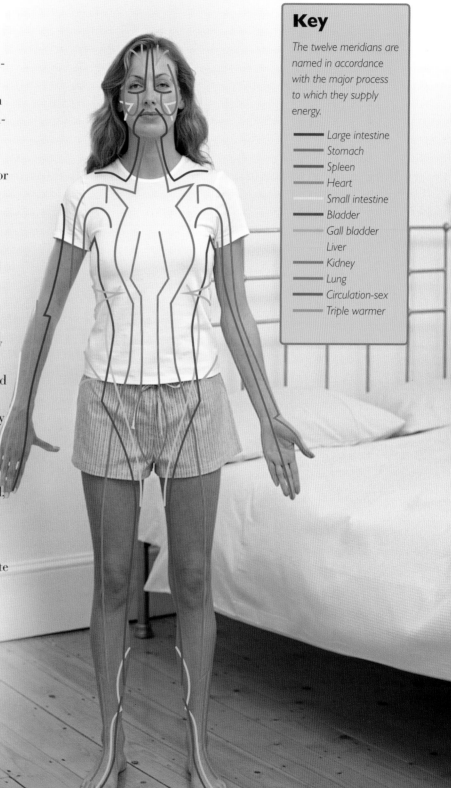

Key

The twelve meridians are named in accordance with the major process to which they supply energy.

— Large intestine
— Stomach
— Spleen
— Heart
— Small intestine
— Bladder
— Gall bladder
— Liver
— Kidney
— Lung
— Circulation-sex
— Triple warmer

Guided meridian
massage

Think of this technique as flushing energy through your meridians in much the same way as you might flush water through a hose pipe. First of all, any blockages or stale energy have to be flushed away by working against the direction of its natural flow. Then fresh energy needs to be encouraged by working in the same direction as its natural flow.

The meridian massage on the following pages makes for a good, strong flow of chi, or life force. Although it may initially sound rather complicated, it is in fact very simple.

You could ask a willing friend or partner to do it for you or you could simply do it yourself. The whole process takes around ten or fifteen minutes and can easily be done over the top of clothing.

To massage the meridians, use either the pads of your fingers, or the palm of your hand – whichever comes more naturally to you. Apply a light pressure and use a firm sweeping movement from one end of section of the meridian line indicated, to the other. This is often referred to as "tracing the line" of the meridian.

The procedure should be done in a relaxed, flowing manner, with the gentle intention of moving energy along the correct pathways. Nothing should be rushed. The mind has a direct influence over the flow of energy, so by really focusing on what you are doing will greatly enhance the effectiveness of the massage. Remember to relax and breathe deeply and fully throughout, and try to minimize the likelihood of any interruptions.

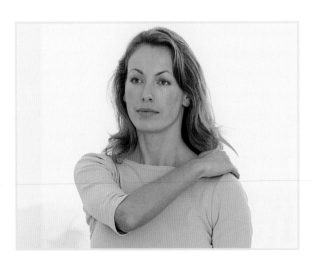

1 *Start at a point midway along your shoulder, about 5cm (2in) down the back of it. Sweep the pads of your middle three fingers in a smooth movement along to your neck, and up the side, ending in the hollow at the base of your skull. Breathe out as you do this. Breathe in to restore your energy and then repeat the process two more times. This is the "flush out" to clear the way for the new flow of energy.*

Now repeat the process in the other direction to renew energy, starting at the hollow in the base of the skull and drawing a line down to the midway point on the shoulder – exhaling as you go. Repeat this movement nine times, breathing in after each sweeping movement to restore energy. Repeat the same process on the other shoulder.

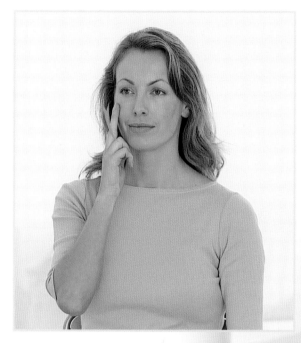

4 Use either the pads of your fingers or the palm of your hand to trace a line up the outside of the shinbone on the out-breath. Start at the ankle and trace the line about an inch away from the shin bone, up to the knee. Repeat a total of three times.

Change direction so that you sweep your hand downward this time on the exhalation, again using the inhalation to restore yourself between strokes. Repeat a total of 9 times.

Then repeat on the other leg.

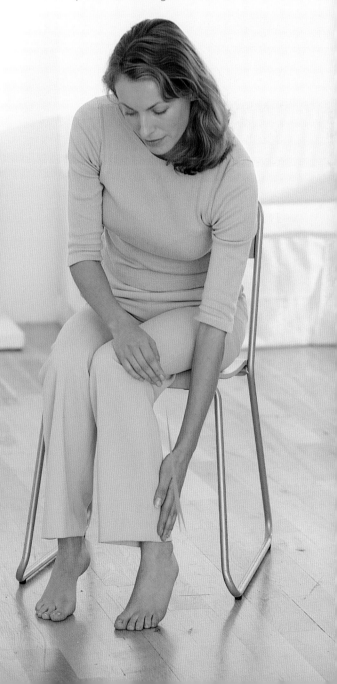

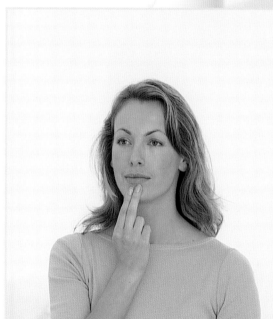

2 Breathing out and starting in the centre of the cheekbone, use either one finger or two to draw a line straight downward, and across to the centre of your chin. Then inhale to restore yourself. Repeat a total of three times.

3 Beginning in the centre of the chin, draw the line along your jaw, and straight up to the centre of the cheekbone, again exhaling as you perform the movement, and inhaling between movements. Repeat a total of nine times.

Then repeat the whole process on the other side of the face.

5 Breathing out, trace a line from the ankle, up the centre back of the calf, to the back of the knee. Inhale to restore your energy. Repeat three times in total.

Now change direction, drawing the energy down from the back of the knee to the ankle on exhalation. Make the sweep smooth, even, and unhurried, and take a deep breath in before each movement. Repeat 9 times.

Repeat on the other leg.

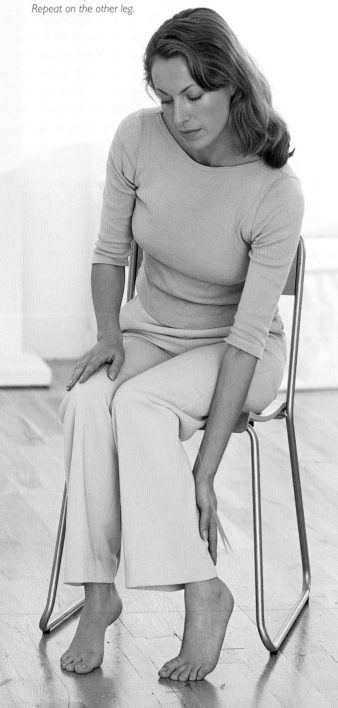

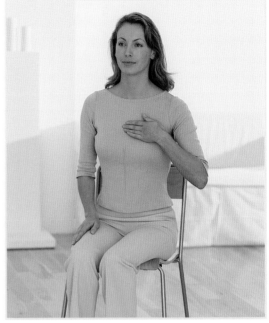

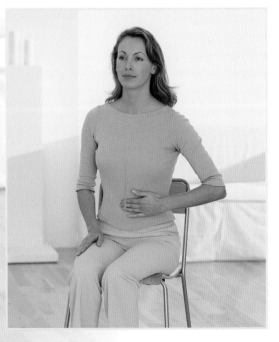

6 Use either the pads of your fingers or the palm of your hand to trace a line from the centre of your ribs (at the base of your breastbone), down your body, to just below the navel. Avoid too much pressure in this area as it may cause feelings of nausea. Repeat three times in total, again exhaling on every movement and inhaling in between.

Reverse the direction, by drawing this centre line upward this time, exhaling as you go, and inhaling to rest. Repeat nine times.

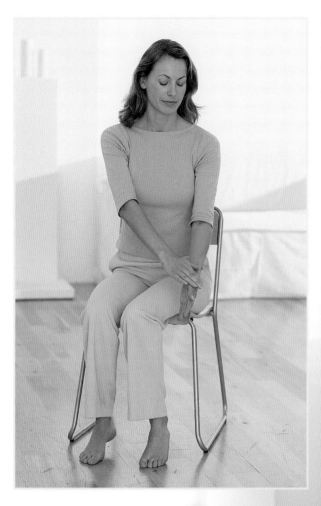

7 Exhaling, trace a line from your thumb up your forearm, to the upper edge of your forearm, above the elbow joint. Repeat a total of three times, inhaling between each movement.

Reverse the direction of this line by sweeping down the forearm to the thumb. Repeat nine times.

...And relax
You should now feel relaxed and revived, but spend a few quiet moments to allow your body's energies to readjust.

Self-massage techniques

The following self-massage techniques can be practised daily as a preventative measure against headaches and migraines, but are equally effective to use as relief during a migraine attack. The techniques do not have to be done as an entire sequence, although they can be done in this way. Feel free to pick and choose from them if you prefer.

2 *Lift your head again to face forward, and using your fingers and heel of one hand, squeeze down the length of your neck and along the ridge of muscle on the top of your shoulder. Repeat several times, or until you experience a feeling of tension being released. Then, do the same along the other shoulder, using whichever hand is comfortable. Continue full abdominal breathing throughout.*

It is be a good idea to try out all the massage techniques on this page the first few times, to observe or even write down any effect they have on you, and then use the ones that you feel are most beneficial to you on a more habitual basis – you can adjust them to meet your ever-changing needs.

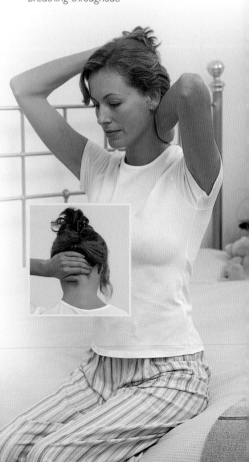

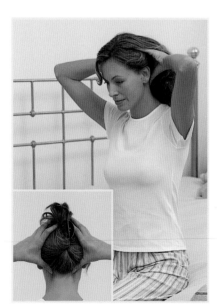

1 *Sit comfortably in an upright chair. Allow your shoulders to sink down and, at the same time, take the pressure off your neck by allowing the crown of your head to float upward toward the ceiling. Draw your chin back a little. Breathe gently and fully into your abdomen, relaxing as much as you can.*

Drop your head down slightly toward your chest. Place your thumbs in the indentations at the base of your skull (on either side of your neck), allowing your fingers to rest comfortably on your head. Massage with your thumbs for a minute or so, using sufficient pressure to produce some sensation. Continue to breathe fully in order to facilitate the flow of energy.

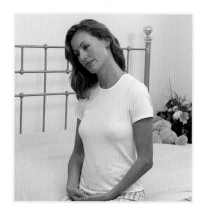

3 *Gently tilt your head to one side, slowly lowering it toward the shoulder. Draw the opposite shoulder down. Then repeat on the other side*

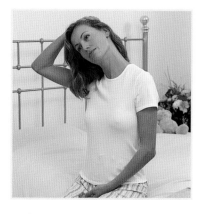

4 *Place your hand on the side of your head and rest it there to provide a feeling of weight. Use your right hand for your right shoulder, and vice versa.*

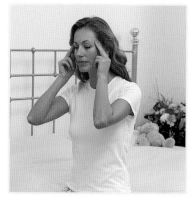

5 *Using the pads of your fingers, gently massage around the temples, using small, circular movements.*

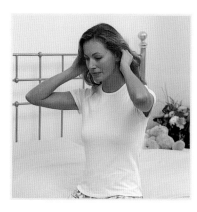

6 *Now gently massage behind your ears, using small, circular movements.*

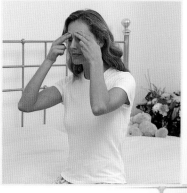

7 *Using small circular movements, massage along the eyebrows, starting at the inner edge. Do both together or one at a time.*

...Release your hands, lifting your head slowly

Relax, and breathe gently for a few moments. Having a drink of water will help the process to continue to work.

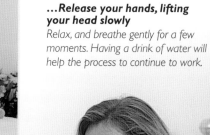

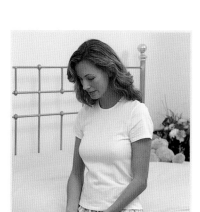

8 *Imagine a thread is tied to your chin, drawing your head down toward your chest. Relax and breathe in this position for a moment or two.*

9 *Interlock your fingers and rest your hands on the back of your head, gently increasing pressure until you experience a comfortable stretch. Continue to breathe.*

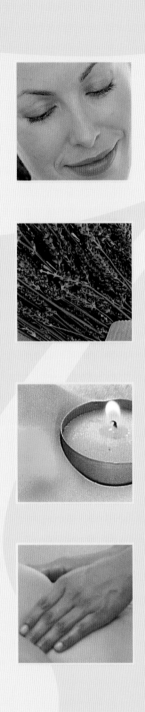

Chapter Seven

Using
ESSENTIAL OILS

Anoint your body,

refresh your spirit,

be guided, drop by aromatic drop,

toward your innermost healing

A gift *from* nature

Essential oils are pure plant extracts, which, as the name suggests, contain the very essence of the plants from which they come. The oils are extracted from the various parts of plants and trees – leaves, flowers, roots, and bark – by distillation, cold-pressing, or solvents. This concentrated essence offers a highly fragranced method of healing.

Although based on ancient wisdom, the use of essential oils as part of holistic healing has really only grown in popularity in the West during the last couple of decades. It is now commonplace to find bottles of aromatic oils in pharmacies and health stores, whereas, previously, they had to be obtained through specialist suppliers. They encourage realignment of the body's energies, helping to eliminate problems such as migraines, and delighting the senses with their many, varied fragrances.

Healing aromas

Our sense of smell is a very powerful thing. We are often quite definite about the smells that we do and don't like, and many aromas can evoke strong memories: transporting us to another time or place, whether our school classroom on a hot summer's afternoon or our parents' garden in springtime.

The fact that scents are so linked to emotions means they play an important role in helping us toward a state of well-being. Learning to use essential oils effectively allows us to choose specific, therapeutic scents for particular situations – whether to stimulate, relax, refresh, energize, send to sleep, or as prevention from debilitating disorders such as migraines.

The active particles in essential oils are so minute that they can enter the bloodstream easily – whether through inhalation or through the surface of the skin, bringing about measurable physiological changes in the body. Aromatic oils can therefore help to harmonize us with our natural forces, balancing us through the layers of mind, body, and spirit, and releasing us from the immense burden of debilitating migraine attacks.

Choosing your oils

There are many therapeutic oils that can help in the relief of migraines. It is important to take care which ones you choose if you are already in the throes of a full-blown migraine attack, as many sense stimulants – aromas included – may prove too invasive at such times and provoke nausea, or even vomiting. If, however, you are aware that an attack feels likely, then it may be successfully averted by using a warm compress of marjoram oil on the back of your neck. Add three drops of marjoram oil to about half a litre (a pint) of hot (not boiling) water, immerse a cloth in it, wring out, and place on the back of the neck. Keep re-immersing in the water as the cloth cools. Reheat the water, if necessary, but do not allow it to boil. Marjoram oil is very pene-trating and will help to relax the muscles and dilate the blood vessels, allowing blood to flow more freely to the brain. A ginger compress would also be effective (see pp. 58–59). Cold compresses using any of the oils on pages 88–89 can also provide relief from congestion headaches. But don't use more than three drops in total to half a litre (a pint) of water. Dip a cloth in the mix-ture, wring out, and place it on the temples, forehead, or back of the neck.

Always be guided by your sense of smell when choosing oils, as different oils are appropriate at different times. Sometimes, you will love a particular aroma and be really drawn to using it, while at other times you may feel an aversion to it and be drawn to try something else. Use this feeling as your internal guide. As you gain the confidence to listen to it, it will become invaluable in revealing the oils that are the most helpful to you and those which are not.

One way of freeing yourself from any preconceived ideas and tapping into your intuition when you are selecting the right oils to help migraine is simply to sweep your hand slowly over a few bottles of oil. You may feel that your hand is "drawn" to a particular one as you explore, or you may have a sense of just "knowing" which one would be best. People have varyingly reported a tingling, a warmth, a coolness, an aversion, or a drawing toward. If you initially select quite a few, repeat the selection process with that smaller group. The more practice you have with this process, the more confidence you will gain in your ability to tune into your body's needs. You will undoubtedly be surprised by how much your body does "know", and this may prove to be a gentle starting point for a further awakening of your senses and intuition.

TRUST YOUR INSTINCTS
Let yourself be drawn to the aromas that you truly love. These will be the ones that eventually do you the most good and help to heal you..

Essential *knowledge*

The essential oils that follow are ones that, generally speaking, will help in the relief of all migraines and headaches. Here, they have been split into three separate categories to help you choose which one might be best at a certain time.

It is important to remember that every individual will react differently to the various oils. It is always worth asking for advice from the staff in your local health store or pharmacy about which oils might best suit your symptoms.

Calming oils

The following oils are most beneficial when you think your migraines stem from nervous tension and exhaustion:

Chamomile: gently fragrant, soothes the spirit, and helps ease the confusion of a troubled mind, bringing about stillness, patience, and understanding

Frankincense: light and exotic, brings a sense of comfort and protection when you are feeling over-burdened and overstretched

Neroli: sweet, fresh fragrance that lifts the burdens of everyday tensions and anxieties, bringing about peace of mind

Lavender: beautifully scented, promotes a sense of gentleness and calm

Bergamot: wonderful, citrus fragrance that lightens the heart, bringing harmony, freshness of spirit, and clarity of mind

Rose: exquisite fragrance, restores a sense of balance, love, and peace

Jasmine: exotic oil, highly prized for its floral scent, captures the essence of femininity, deeply balancing for people exhausted by the stresses of "power living"

Benzoin: warmly aromatic fragrance, gives a sense of comfort and protection while calming the senses

Stimulating oils

The following oils are useful when you have a congestion-related headache and need clarity:

Ginger: warm, zesty smell, awakens the senses, bringing a sense of strength

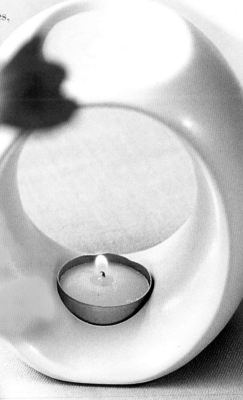

BURN BABY BURN
Burning essential oils in a specially designed oil burner is a great way to infuse your surroundings with healing aromas.

Juniper: fragrant, woody aroma, gives clear awakening and vitality

Marjoram: herby and slightly bitter-smelling, encourages the dilation of blood vessels, bringing healing to congested areas

Rosemary: sharp and woody aroma, clears the mind and is reputed to improve the memory, facilitating concentration and releasing emotional clutter

Peppermint: fresh and clear, helps rid the body of lethargy, encouraging renewed energy

Spearmint: slightly sweeter-smelling than peppermint, stimulates the mind to assist with clear thinking

Hormone-balancing oils

The following oils are helpful if your migraines may be linked to your menstrual cycle:

Rose: has a particular affinity with the female reproductive system, purifies and regulates, helping to relieve depression caused by hormonal imbalances

Jasmine: a valuable uterine tonic, helps to relieve menstrual pains, cramps, and migraines

Geranium: heady, floral scent, a great tonic for the kidneys, helps to relieve water retention, regulate the hormonal cycle, calm irritation, and relieve depression

Sweet Fennel: sharp aniseed aroma, has a particular affinity with the female reproductive system, almost mimicking oestrogen, which makes it useful for dispelling fluid retention and pre-menstrual syndrome

Using essential oils

There are many ways to enjoy using essential oils. A few drops can be added to a hot bath as a special treat for the senses, oil can be burned in an oil burner (see left) to enhance surroundings with a healing scent, compresses can be made (see pp. 58–59 and 86–87), a few drops can be dabbed on a handkerchief to use when you feel the need, or the oils can be applied directly onto the skin during a relaxing massage (see pp. 90–91).

Ideally, you should incorporate essential oils into your regular routine, perhaps taking an aromatic bath three or four times a week or having a weekly massage to keep you feeling calm, healthy, and in balance. Refer to the list of essential oils on the left to decide which ones are most suitable for you, bearing in mind that your needs will undoubtedly vary with time – so be prepared to be flexible in your choices.

Essential oils can be used singly or mixed together, but for reasons of safety, if being used in massage, should be diluted in a base oil (called the "carrier" oil) – about five or six drops in total to a tablespoon of carrier.

The main thing is to really relish and enjoy using these healing oils, and also to take pleasure in the reawakening of your sense of smell. Your initial attitude to them – in terms of whether or not you truly believe in their power – will have a

A Word of Warning

Although essential oils are natural and can be very good for you, they can build up to toxic levels in the body if used too frequently, so must be used with respect. If you use them regularly, have a complete break every now and again, perhaps one week out of every four. If you are in any doubt as to the usage of a particular oil, or the frequency with which it can be safely used, it is advisable to seek advice from a qualified aromatherapist. It is also important to keep essential oils out of the reach of children.

direct bearing on how beneficial they are for you personally. This is because the intent behind what we set out to do will determine the outcome. We have the choice as to whether to close ourselves down to something or open ourselves up to it. In order to achieve – and direct – the flow of energy required for optimal health, we have to have an attitude of open assimilation when we set out to discover the many wonderful properties of essential oils. So enjoy experimenting with them and benefiting from their immense healing properties.

Healing oil *massage*

Massage using essential oil diluted in a carrier oil, such as grapeseed or almond oil, is a very effective and pleasurable way of treating the body and bringing about a state of balance, relaxation, and healing. There is nothing more wonderful than a deep but gentle body massage from a sensitive therapist or friend to bring about a state of well-being, and the use of therapeutic essential oils makes this all the more effective.

Tension and stress can be greatly relieved by regular massage, as can aches, pains, and muscle fatigue. Regular massage of the neck and shoulders can help enormously in the relief and prevention of chronic headaches and migraines and can greatly help toward improving the circulation. This state of well-being is a very sound platform from which to bring yourself into a feeling of balance, health, and a migraine-free existence.

Simple back & shoulder massage

★ Set aside 20 to 30 minutes and choose a suitable space for the massage. Make sure you are warm and comfortable, and then lie on your front. Candles and soothing music create a relaxing atmosphere. Select your essential oils – usually a maximum of three – and dilute in a suitable carrier oil, such as sweet almond or grapeseed. Use six drops of essential oil to one tablespoon of carrier oil. Remove clothing from your upper body, which should be covered with warm towels before the massage

begins. This helps to relax the muscles, releasing superficial tension and making the body more receptive to the treatment. There is no need for the "masseur" to be too concerned about using any particular techniques. Giving and receiving touch is a natural human interaction, so they should just be led by their intuition, using the following information as guidelines:

★ Firstly use the flat palms of both hands to press the lower back, up each side of the spine in turn, to the shoulders.

★ Remove the towel and spread the oils over the surface of the back, using large, circular movements. Spend time working the oils into the muscles, with further circular movements.

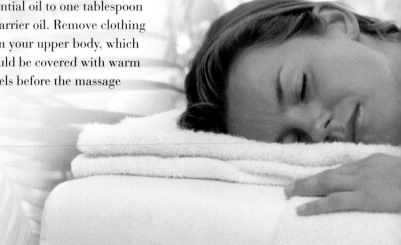

★ Work your way gradually up to the shoulders. Be prepared to spend time working on the muscles here, as this is the seat of much of the tension that causes migraines. Use gentle kneading or squeezing actions with the fingertips and heel of the hand.

★ Now work your way up each side of the neck, using small circular movements with your thumbs and the tips of your fingers. Proceed with caution, as the neck is a sensitive and complex area.

★ Many headaches can be alleviated by massaging the indentations at the base of the skull. Use circular movements with the thumbs, resting the fingers on the head for support.

★ Still using circular movements, now massage the scalp, aiming to create movement in the skin over the top of the bony structure of the skull. This increases the blood flow and thus alleviates congestion headaches.

★ Finish the soothing massage by using flowing, circular movements down the back again. Then place one hand on the "patient's" neck and the other hand on the base of their spine. Relax for a few full, deep breaths. Remove your hands when you feel ready and cover the receiver with a warm towel again. Both of you should then take a little time to relax, and to drink some water.

THE HEALING TOUCH
Regular soothing massages from a friend or bodywork therapist can help immensely toward relieving, or maybe even completely preventing, headaches and migraines.

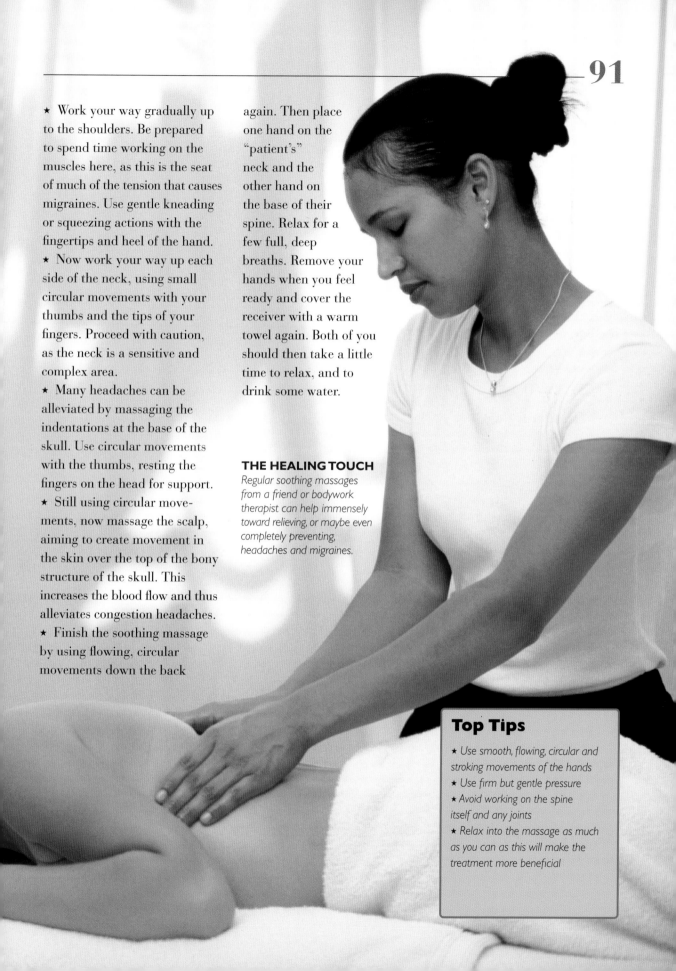

Top Tips

★ *Use smooth, flowing, circular and stroking movements of the hands*
★ *Use firm but gentle pressure*
★ *Avoid working on the spine itself and any joints*
★ *Relax into the massage as much as you can as this will make the treatment more beneficial*

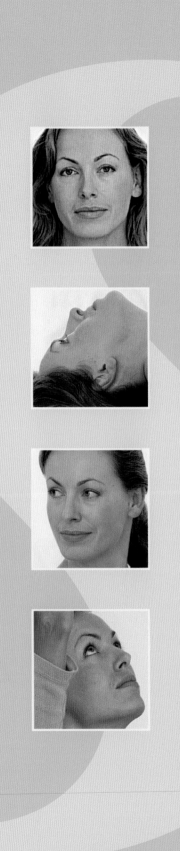

Chapter Eight

EXERCISING
your way to health

Exercise your body well and with care,

move forward into the world with ease,

for your body is your own creation,

sacred home to your eternal spirit

The *importance* of exercise

When you are struggling with a throbbing headache or in the throes of a heavy migraine attack, the last thing on your mind is likely to be exercise. However, gentle exercise is of paramount importance as it helps both your body and your mind become more supple.

Gentle exercise promotes an increase in your energy levels, boosting your emotional feelings and often helping to dispel the kind of everyday stresses and anxieties that contribute to complaints like migraines.

If you can feel a migraine threatening, you can often stop it in its tracks by having a good stretch, taking half a dozen deep breaths, and going for a brisk walk. Regular exercise is therefore very helpful to people trying to cope with, and alleviate, the pain and stresses of headaches and migraine attacks.

Exercise your chi
It is believed by alternative health practitioners that poor health, including conditions such as migraines, are an indication of unevenly distributed personal energy flow. Disciplines like tai chi and yoga – from which the exercises in the following pages are drawn – help to improve health by increasing and redistributing energies evenly throughout the body. They offer an opportunity to experience the connection between different aspects of your being, combining spiritual awareness with discipline of the mind and the physical body. The gentle movements and stretches can be modified to suit all fitness levels.

Natural patterns
You may notice that your body's physical capabilities and the quality of energy flow vary from time to time. This is because we are not only affected by the more obvious factors, such as lifestyle, pressures of work, and everyday responsibilities, but we also respond to natural forces, such as the turn of the seasons and the phases of the moon. There are times of strong forces, the most obvious one being the fullness of springtime, with its rapid new growth. Conversely, there is less natural energy available during winter, making it a time for more reflective, introspective pursuits.

By remembering that you are part of this natural flow of life, you will feel more at peace with the changes – and problems – that are an intrinsic part of your life. Be guided by the ebbs and flows of the changing energy and by how you are feeling. By learning to recognize your ups

There is merit in both activity and stillness; together, they produce balance.

and downs you will be able to start to work with them. If you are the sort of person who is either "up in the clouds" or "down in the depths", regular exercise will help enormously to even out these swings, which can bring about violent migraines. It can be difficult to discipline yourself into a regular exercise plan. However, you will really feel the benefits, so do persist.

Remembering, too, that life itself is neutral and that it is our own emotions that produce "good" or "bad" feelings may give you a more balanced perception. Life is not something that is "done" to you, but rather, something that you experience according to your own choices.

Exercise programme

The exercises that follow are based mainly on the principles of Chinese yoga, which teaches the importance of keeping the body's movements fluid, in order to enhance the energy flow. It advises against over-stretching or "holding" any posture in tension as this would inhibit the flow of chi. The principle is that if you listen to, and work within, the limitations of your body, you can gradually extend those limitations, strengthening the body, and encouraging balance between all aspects – mind, body, and spirit. Your progress should then be quite rapid, as the body will not be forced to recover from stiffness or injuries imposed by pushing it too far.

All the exercises suggested have a positive effect on the spine, neck, and shoulders – areas that so often carry the tension causing migraines. The exercises can be practised daily, but should be done at least twice weekly to feel the benefits. They can be followed in sequence, or if you have only a little time or feel a particular benefit of one or two of them, a "dip-in-dip out" approach is fine – guided by your own changing needs and preferences. Even ten or fifteen minutes a day, or half an hour a few times a week, is enough to bring about an improvement.

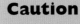

Caution

If your migraines stem from musculo-skeletal problems, such as a displacement or injury to your back or neck, caution is advisable. You should continue to follow the advice of your health practitioner as to which form of exercise is right for you.

You will find yourself becoming wonderfully supple as the chi starts to circulate freely, bringing strength, relaxation, restored balance, and freedom from – or a reduction in – migraines.

It is important to approach the exercises with a sense of focus. Set aside some time as sacred for alleviating your headaches. Wear loose and comfortable clothes, and make sure that your work area is warm and free from clutter. The aim is to provide yourself with a sense of clarity and peace, which – with practice – can become so much a part of you, that you will carry this attitude with you throughout your daily activities.

Each exercise is presented in three phases. The first phase is "the starting position"; the second "the sequence" – gentle movements timed to fit with your breathing; and the third "the extension" – taking the movement into more of a stretch. However, you should always warm up (see pp. 96–97) before starting the exercises themselves.

Warming *up*

It is always important to give some time and attention to "warming up" the body before attempting any exercises. This not only introduces gentle movement to your muscles and joints, encouraging the blood to start flowing and the body to awaken, but it also sets the scene for more specific exercises, allowing the mind time to "tune in" and start to work with your body.

2 LOOSEN UP THE HIPS

Stand with your feet shoulder-width apart, your knees slightly bent, and your hands placed lightly on your hips. Circle the hips six times in each direction, using your hands to help you.

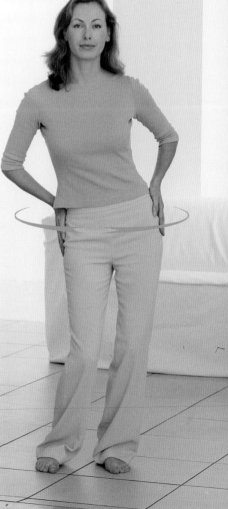

The more you involve your mind in the following exercises, the more benefit you will gain; the ideal is for all to work as one – mind, body, and spirit.

It is best to do the warm-up exercises in the order in which they are presented. They, like the exercises to come, are based on Chinese yoga and tai chi movements, and therefore provide a good foundation from which to explore the exercises themselves (see pp. 98–107).

1 GENTLY STRETCH THE NECK

Gently tilt your head to the side, moving your ear down toward your shoulder to give your neck a nice stretch. Repeat six times on each side, making sure that you do not over-strain.

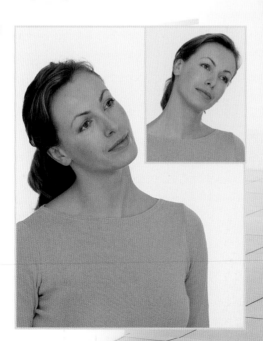

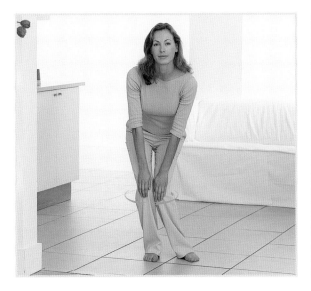

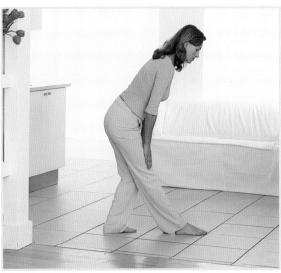

3 FREE THE KNEES

Bend your knees slightly, bend forward, and place your hands on your knees. Use your hands to circle the knees six times in one direction and six times in the other. If you have any problems with your knees, it is best to avoid this exercise.

4 HAMSTRING STRETCH

Extend one foot about a single pace in front of you, keeping your heel down, and bend your back leg. Place both hands – one on top of the other – just above the knee of the extended leg. You will have to bend over slightly in order to do this. Raise the toes of the front foot as far as is comfortable and lean into your hands, only using a comfortable pressure. You should experience a wonderful stretch up the back of your leg while in this position, which is called the "monkey stance" in Chinese yoga. Repeat this up to six times on each side.

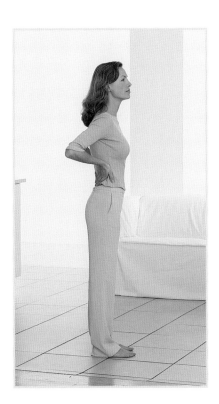

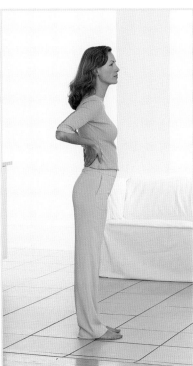

5 BALLOON BREATHING

Stand with your legs about hip-width apart, place your hands on your kidney area (lower back), fingers pointing downward, and breathe deeply into your abdomen.

As you breathe in through your nose, feel your abdomen expanding. You can use the image of a balloon inflating to help you.

As you breathe out through your mouth, gently contract the abdomen, using the image of a balloon deflating to help you.

Repeat for several breaths. Start with three or four breaths, and increase to a maximum of twelve inhalations and exhalations as you become more comfortable. Guard against strenuous over-breathing, however, as this may make you feel rather dizzy.

The *flexing* of the *bow*

The spine can become inflexible through incorrect posture or under-use, leading to muscular tension and restriction of movement. And such stiffness in the spine, neck, and shoulders is a common cause of migraines. This exercise can help greatly in the relief of headaches of this nature.

The "flexing of the bow" is of particular benefit to people who suffer from habitual stiffness in the spine and shoulder area. It will also help nourish the nervous system, bringing relief from nervous headaches. It can be a useful exercise to practise at the onset of a headache or migraine that results from stiffness in the muscles – perhaps from too many hours driving or sitting behind a desk. However, it is also a useful exercise to keep the spine, neck, and shoulders generally more flexible and open, which could mean less migraine symptoms in the first place. It is therefore advisable to practise it on a regular basis, if possible.

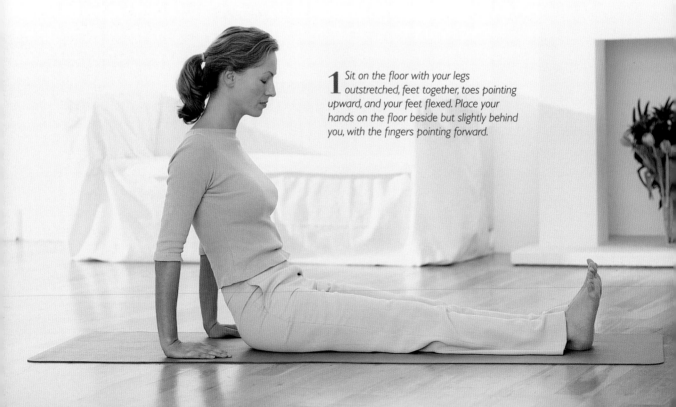

1 Sit on the floor with your legs outstretched, feet together, toes pointing upward, and your feet flexed. Place your hands on the floor beside but slightly behind you, with the fingers pointing forward.

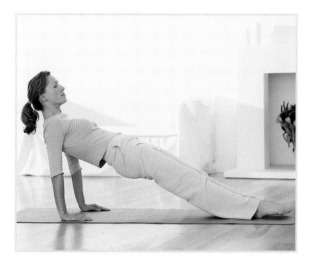

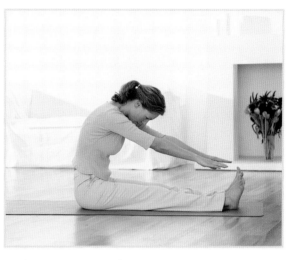

2 As you breathe in, start to lean the weight of the body back on to your hands and arms, lifting your hips, and keeping your legs straight. Your head should keep looking forward and your shoulders should not hunch.

3 As soon as your body forms a straight (diagonal) line, start to lower the hips back down to the floor on the out-breath, reaching forward toward your toes for an effective counterstretch. It does not matter if you can't reach your toes – have the feeling that you are reaching forward out of your hips and try to extend your chest. Repeat steps 1 and 2 up to nine times.

EXTENSION

Only progress to this extension when you feel completely confident in this movement.

4 Repeat the movement in step 1 again on the in-breath, but this time gently drop your head back and point your toes down toward the floor when you have your hips raised off the floor.

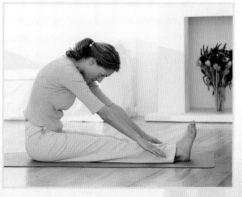

5 Start to release the position on the out-breath as before, bringing your hips down, but this time flex the feet as you bend forward toward the toes, producing a good stretch down the back of the legs. Repeat steps 3 and 4, with care, up to nine times.

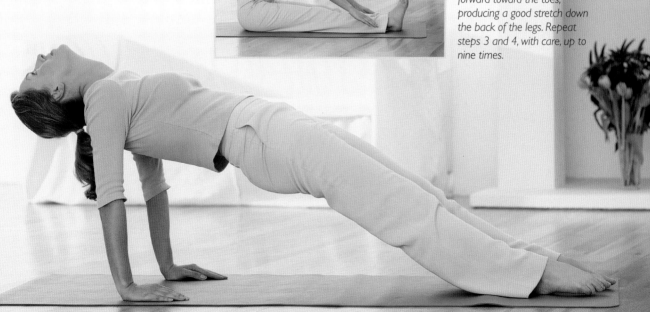

The *praying mantis* awakens

This simple exercise encourages fluidity in the spine, which gently awakens the nervous system, allowing your natural energy to flow more strongly, and releasing any emotional and/or physical tensions and restrictions that may be causing your migraines.

vitality at the same time. It is of particular benefit at times when your back is feeling "stuck" or "locked", and it will encourage a feeling of fluidity and elongation, ridding the body of that hunched-up feeling that so often accompanies migraines. This exercise is a very good rejuvenator following a migraine attack. Use the image of a snake to encourage your spine toward ease of movement.

This exercise improves the flexibility of the entire spine and neck, strengthening the muscles and increasing your sense of

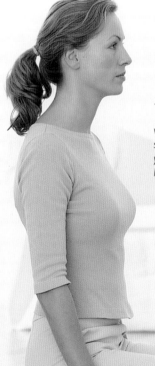

1 Kneel on the floor, sitting on your feet, with your neck and shoulders relaxed, and your arms hanging loosely by your sides.

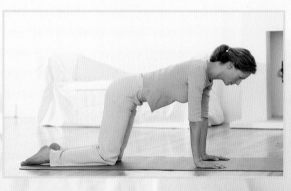

2 Breathing in, move your body forward until you are on all-fours, with your hands under your shoulders, your back in a straight (horizontal) line, and your head forward.

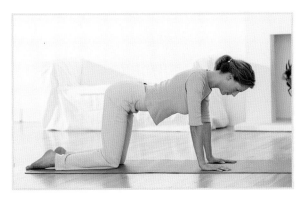

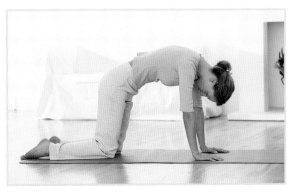

3 Breathing out, begin to hollow your back and lower your stomach toward the floor.
Breathing in, return your back to neutral.

4 Breathing out, scoop your stomach up and arch your spine – keep your head in a neutral position, looking down. Breathing in, return to neutral.
While breathing out, sit back on your heels. Repeat the whole sequence carefully up to nine times, depending on how feel.

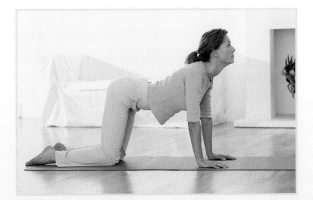

EXTENSION

Only when you are completely comfortable with the sequence should you move into this extension.

5 As you lower your stomach and hollow your back in step 2, lift your chin so that you are looking up, but be very careful not to strain your neck.

6 As you arch the back in step 3, tighten the stomach muscles and tuck the chin toward the chest. Do up to nine repetitions of steps 5 and 6.

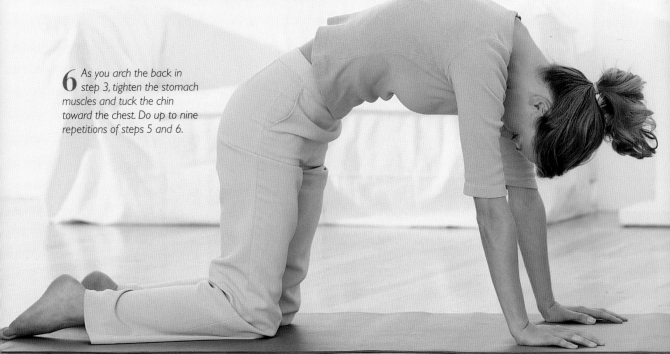

The eagle looks from east to west

The more the body, and in particular the spinal area, can be encouraged to move, the less likely it is that stresses and tensions will accumulate, leading to migraines. This twisting exercise promotes flexibility in and freedom of movement in the spine.

Tension and stress often accumulate in the lower back, leading to feelings of being overburdened by life and producing "heavy" headaches.

This exercise encourages a flexible and nourishing twist along the spine, particularly around the waist and lower back, alleviating such tension.

Caution

Take care, however, not to over-twist the spine – especially if you are not used to exercising this area. The twist explained below also works the hips, so again exercise caution if your hips are at all stiff.

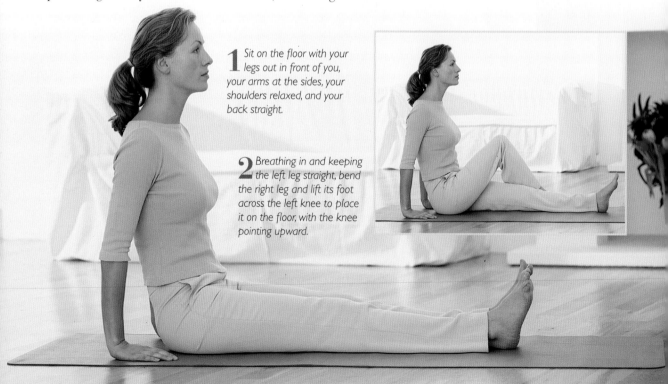

1 *Sit on the floor with your legs out in front of you, your arms at the sides, your shoulders relaxed, and your back straight.*

2 *Breathing in and keeping the left leg straight, bend the right leg and lift its foot across the left knee to place it on the floor, with the knee pointing upward.*

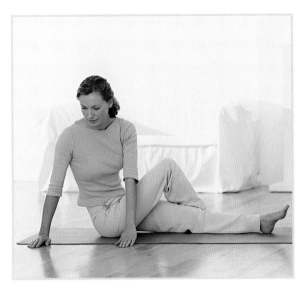

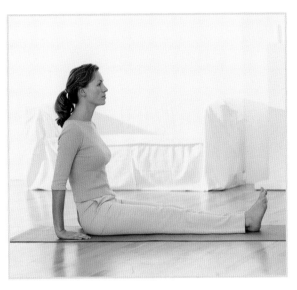

3 Breathing out and keeping your back upright and your right hand on the floor behind you for support, take your left hand across to the right side of your body, and place it on the floor beside your right hip.

Breathing in, untwist the top half of your body, returning to face centre.

4 Breathing out, extend your right leg on the floor in order to repeat steps 1–3 on the other side, bending the left leg and twisting to the left. Build up to six repetitions on each side.

EXTENSION

Only attempt the extension if your body is entirely comfortable with the sequence above. Make sure you allow the breath to come and go naturally as you do it.

5 Begin as before, bringing your right leg across your left knee, but this time take your left arm over the top of your right knee, anchoring the palm of your left hand against the outside of your left knee. This arm can then act as a lever, enabling you to extend the stretch toward the right. The right arm acts as a support behind you – the fingers pointing backward.

As with all these exercises, just begin to release and return to the starting position as you reach a point of extension – before the stretch becomes a strain. Then repeat on the other side and gradually build up to six repetitions on each side of the body.

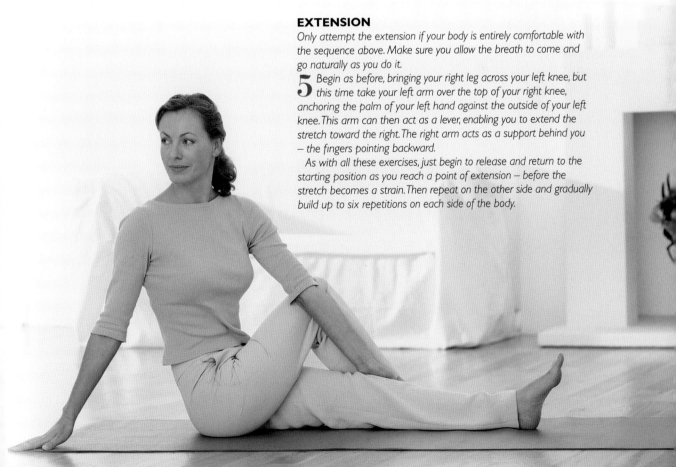

The *cobra* raises *its* head

Poor posture is a symptom of our sedentary, often desk-bound, modern culture. If practised regularly, the following exercise will help prevent slumping shoulders and under-used back and stomach muscles, bringing relief from postural headaches.

This exercise will release tension that has built up in the spine and neck through poor posture, which often leads to headaches. It will also exercise and nourish the digestive system, helping to alleviate migraines that may result from overloaded or inefficient digestion. Do not attempt to do this exercise immediately after eating; wait at least an hour or two.

1 Lie face down on the floor, with your forehead resting on the floor and your elbows bent so that your hands are right beside your shoulders.

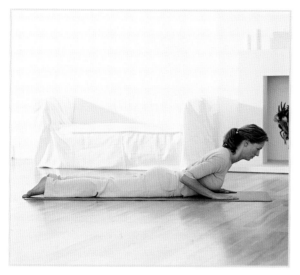

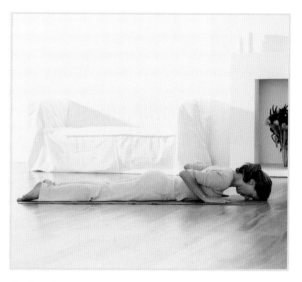

2 Breathing in, point the toes, and – keeping the back as relaxed as you can – lift the chest and head off the floor to look forward. Keep your weight forward as much as you can, using your arms rather than the back muscles. Draw the shoulder blades back toward the centre of the spine. Make sure that the hands are directly under the shoulders, and do not over-stretch.

3 Breathing out, use your arms to lower your forehead to the floor once again, thus returning to the starting position. Repeat up to nine times, but take care to relax your back throughout and not to strain your neck.

EXTENSION

If you feel comfortable with the sequence, progress to the extension, again breathing in a relaxed manner throughout.

4 Repeat steps 1 and 2 but this time, as you push up, try to straighten your arms, being careful not to lock or hyperextend them. Also lift your chin to look up.

When you feel you have reached a comfortable limit, ease off, and return to the starting position. Relax completely between repetitions.

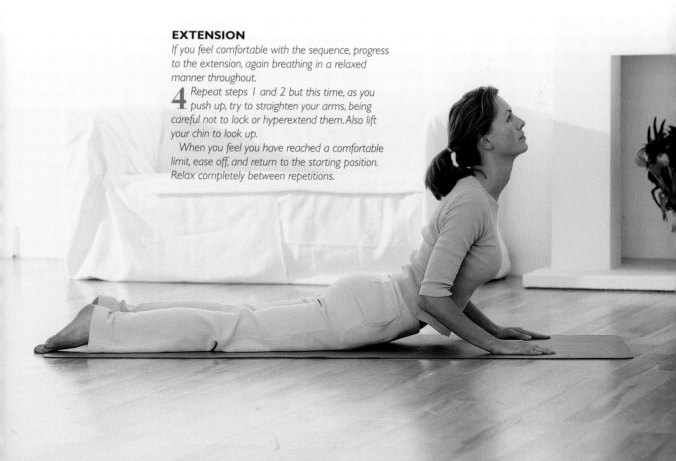

Paying homage *to the* *universe*

This sequence of movements gently exercises the whole body, flexing and stretching both the front of the torso and the back. This is an ideal routine to perform first thing in the morning, as it gently awakens the entire body.

The major benefits of this exercise – apart from being a real pleasure to perform – are to the digestive and nervous systems. When these are out of balance, they can be significant factors in the development of nauseous headaches and migraines. In working through the sequence, you may find it helpful to use the image of flowing through the different movements as light flows into darkness and as darkness recedes into light.

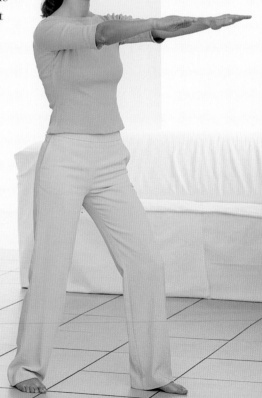

2 *Breathing in, step forward a pace with your left foot, bend your knee, and sweep your arms forward to shoulder height.*

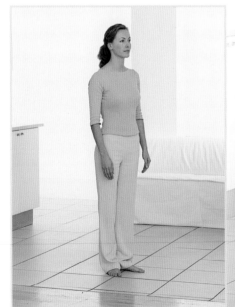

1 *Stand with your heels together, your body upright but relaxed, and your hands hanging loosely by your sides: the "eagle stance".*

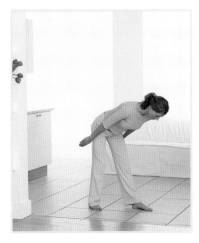

3 *Breathing out, take the weight on to the back leg and bend it while straightening the front leg. At the same time, sweep your arms down to your sides, or slightly behind, while you bend your body forward – the spine following a natural sweeping curve.*

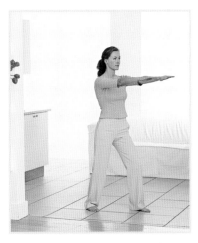

4 *Breathing in, bring the weight forward on to the front leg again, and sweep your arms back up to shoulder height.*

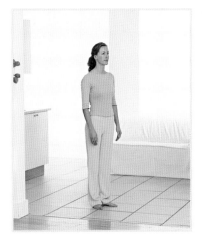

5 *Breathing out, return to the starting position. Repeat but this time with your right foot forward.*
Then, repeat steps 1–3 up to nine times on each side, trying to maintain a fluid feeling throughout the sequence.

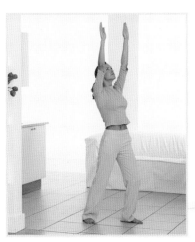

EXTENSION

Only progress to this extension when you feel confident about the sequence above. Breathing should remain relaxed throughout.

6 *As you step forward, bending the knee, sweep the arms right up above your head and look up. Try to keep your weight forward over your front foot, but be careful of your balance.*

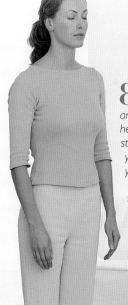

7 *Taking your weight on to the back foot, swing both arms down and back and at the same time bend forward; you should be looking at your knees. Your arms are now extended backward and upward away from your head.*

8 *Bringing your weight forward again, sweep your arms back up above your head, and then return to the starting position – drawing your foot back in, and resting your arms at your sides.*
Repeat steps 5–7 up to six times on alternate sides, with a feeling of one fluid movement into the next, throughout the exercise.

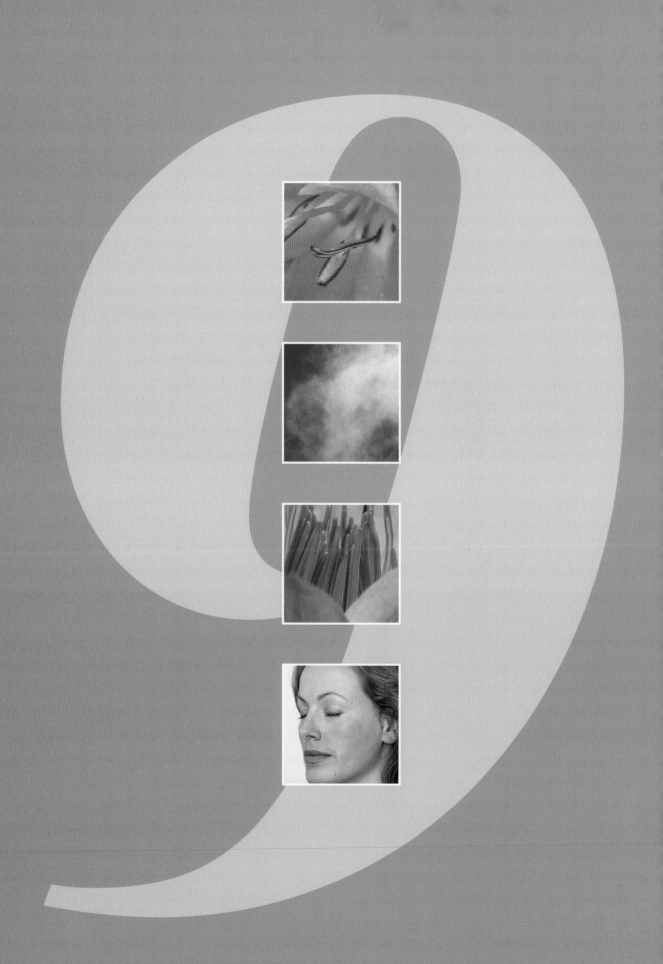

Chapter Nine

Healing with
COLOUR

Let sunlight dance with raindrops

and cast its arc of colour across

the heavens — be inspired

The *power of* *colour*

We are strongly influenced in our daily lives by the cycles of light and darkness and by the many colours that surround us. And colours, in the same way as aromas, can provoke strong emotional responses in us. We often find ourselves being drawn to particular colours, wanting to wear them or to introduce them into our surroundings in some way.

We may find that we react quite markedly to some colours, perhaps being calmed by blues and mauves or stimulated by the reds and oranges of autumn. And we may find that we "go off" certain colours periodically and have a complete change of colour scheme. This is our instinctive way of noticing the changes taking place within us. The use of colour could be thought of as our own emotional language, providing a direct link to the flow of colour in our energy field, or aura. When illness, such as a migraine, is experienced it indicates a lack of flow of this natural energy or highlights an imbalance in our natural "chakra colours" (see pp. 114–115).

Colour through time

Before the onset of technology as we know it, advanced cultures lived their lives very much more in tune with nature and the subtle energies of life than most of us do today. They therefore developed an in-depth knowledge of the importance of colours and

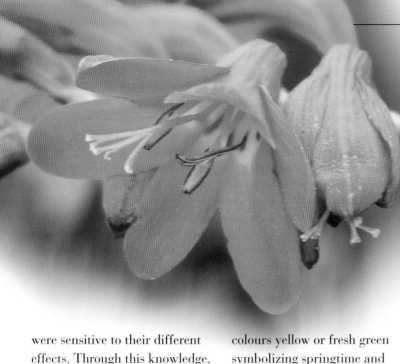

were sensitive to their different effects. Through this knowledge, they were able to develop methods of colour healing based on the specific benefits that each colour can bring. The ancient Egyptians used clear quartz crystals to split natural sunlight into the colours of the spectrum and then directed these pure colours to various areas, where people could go to absorb their vibrations to promote healing and well-being.

Although much of this ancient knowledge has been lost to us, we still attach a lot of meaning to certain colours: we see the colours yellow or fresh green symbolizing springtime and rebirth, pink indicating love, purple being worn as ceremonial robes or for formal ritual, and white conveying purity or a state of enlightenment, for example.

Colour, colour everywhere

The world is bursting with ever-changing colours, and, as you become more aware of them, more open to their individual and varied energies and vibrations, you will start to feel their different effects on your state of being. By failing to notice what is around us, we close down and become desensitized to their properties.

By learning to acknowledge and use our senses more fully, we begin to open ourselves up to the more subtle messages around us, bringing about a more peaceful state of mind – a feeling of being more connected to the natural world.

Feelings of being "disconnected" can lead to stress and feelings of anxiety, which can lead directly to headaches and migraines. But when you feel "connected", these tensions no longer have a place in your life, so open your eyes fully to the amazing colours in nature. You can find colours even on a grey winter's day: the changing, subtle shades of the sky, the incredibly beautiful colours of the trees, the mixed tones of the bark, the bright greens of moss and lichens. Nature is very colourful through all the seasons of the year, but at times, you have to take the time to look more carefully to truly appreciate it. Learning to pay attention will reward you with myriad gifts.

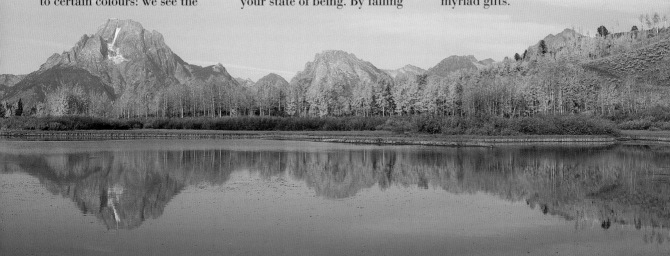

The *energy* of colour

Every individual's energy field is made up of subtle vibrations. What's more, every colour also has its own vibrational properties, which can be absorbed into the body through our energy field with wide-ranging effects. Everyone responds to different colours individually according to whether their own "vibration" is in tune with that of the colours.

While some people are able to see or sense auras, or energetic bodies, in the form of colours or light around the human body, most of us cannot. However, we are more energetically aware than we perhaps realize. We constantly respond to the messages around us, including those given off by different colours. For example, we often feel strongly about whether or not to buy and wear clothes of a certain colour or which colour to decorate our house in. We are also often instinctively aware of the energetic state of those around us, finding that we can "read" one another's feelings and "colour of mood" quite well. This sensitivity can be used to our benefit when introducing a colour with the intention of rebalancing and healing our own energy field, thus relieving ourselves from the pain and frustration of migraines.

Colour associations

Let us look a little more closely at the colours used to describe people's emotional states. If we declare that a person is "green with envy", for example, we are tuning into an imbalance of heart energy at that time. This is because the colour green is associated with the heart centre being in a state of harmony and balance. When this becomes disrupted by feelings of envy and jealousy, a sludgy green is likely to emerge in the energy field. And if the feelings are very strong, the green will be almost black and will most certainly feel unpleasant. Balance in this area, on the other hand, will be revealed as a bright, fresh green in the aura. Someone who is full of love for others will radiate a glowing pink colour, which feels wonderful to be around, as it spreads positive vibrations.

Melancholy reveals itself as the colour blue in the energy field and radiates a sense of feeling "blue". If someone is feeling intensely bad tempered and thwarted by life, we are aware that they are carrying a black cloud with them – they are in a "black" mood – the message is to stay well away from them.

On the whole, if a colour is sludgy or jarring, it is revealing an imbalance, whereas if it is clear and beautiful, it signifies a state of balance.

Colour therapy

Colour can be absorbed in many ways for the purposes of healing – through the eyes, the skin, and also through our energy centres, thereby enabling the whole being to be flooded with colour. The innate intelligence of the body will then direct the colour to where it is most needed to bring about balance, helping to release blockages within the energy field. These blockages may exist for many reasons, but, once they have been released and a sense of equilibrium has been restored, then many physical, mental, and emotional conditions, including migraine, will be greatly alleviated.

Enjoy experimenting with and using the myriad effects of different colours. Open yourself to the subtleties of using them therapeutically and you will wonder how you could have missed it all before.

With the red ray I walk with strength and vitality along my chosen path in life.

With the warmth of the orange ray I am able to fulfil my creativity with joy and vitality.

With the clarity of the yellow ray I can think clearly and I am open to new possibilities.

The harmony of green allows me to trust in the flow of life, enabling me to feel balance and compassion.

With the cooling blue ray, I can release tension and allow myself to relax, bringing me peace with myself and those around me.

The indigo ray brings positive, happy thoughts, bringing with it calm and quiet intuition.

With the spiritual connection of magenta, I am able to give freely of the abundance I draw to me.

Chakras & *colour*

The body has seven major energy centres, or chakras, as they are known in ancient Indian philosophy – each of which relates to a different energy and colour. These chakras are spinning areas of energy, which give and receive subtle information, and are positioned at intervals in a vertical formation from the base of the spine up to the crown of the head.

The chakras are visible or tangible only to some healers and clairvoyants, who learn to interpret what they can indicate in terms of a person's health.

Each of the chakras are sensitive and responsive to a particular colour vibration. If all the chakras are in a healthy and open condition, all the related colours will be present in equal measure in the energy field, or aura. However, this is often not the case, as various chakras may become blocked, diminished, or even temporarily closed down, resulting in the corresponding colours being "missing" from a person's energy field.

As well as relating to a specific colour, each chakra relates to a different body function, so if there is a problem in the energy flow, either in a particular chakra or in the connections between them, this will be experienced as mental, emotional, or physical disturbances, such as migraine.

Balancing the chakras

An understanding of the chakras, combined with the knowledge of how they are linked to our physical health, can give us a picture of how important it is to keep them in a state of balance. As we learn colour therapy techniques, we are likely to experience changes in our emotional and mental elements, as well as in the initial physical complaint we set out to address, because these aspects of ourselves are inextricably linked. If we learn about what each chakra represents (see pp. 115–117), we will equip ourselves with the knowledge to try to figure out which of our chakras may be out of balance at any given time. We can then use the relevant colour or colours to start the healing process.

People who suffer from migraine attacks or headaches often show an imbalance in the third eye chakra (see p. 117), which can be due to constantly rushing thoughts and an over-intellectual take on life.

The following colours are often helpful when dealing with or trying to avoid migraines. *Violet* is a useful colour to use as it helps to clear and still the mind, encouraging valuable insights and a deeper wisdom. *Blue* is a good colour to use as it is soothing for stress and tension around the neck and shoulders, as well as for headaches associated with emotional turbulence or mental overload. Blue is also soothing for feverish headaches and inflammation. **Yellow** can be used with great effect for the nauseous "liverish" feeling that can sometimes accompany migraine attacks, as it stimulates the digestive process and helps clear away any feelings of sluggishness. **Orange** is a useful colour if migraine attacks are linked with the menstrual cycle, as this is the colour with the most affinity to the female reproductive system.

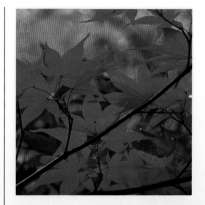

CROWN CHAKRA
Cooperation, service, self-confidence

THIRD EYE CHAKRA
Love, joy, deep awareness

THROAT CHAKRA
Intuition, truth, loyalty

HEART CHAKRA
Balance, trust

SOLAR PLEXUS CHAKRA
Intelligence, aspiration, courage

SACRAL CHAKRA
Sexuality, creativity, expression

BASE CHAKRA
Survival, action, drive, will

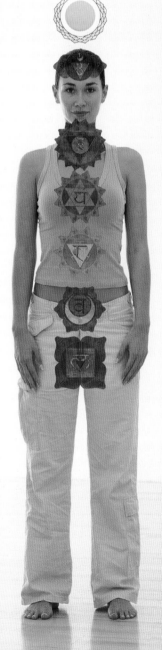

THE SEVEN CHAKRAS
Each of the seven chakras is a certain colour, with its own vibration and its own emotional effects, as well as physical ones.

The base chakra: red

This centre is located at the base of the spine, relates to the legs, feet, base of the spine, blood, and bones, and vibrates at the frequency of the colour red.

It is the seat of our male energy: our drive and commitment to survival. Through this centre, we feel a connection to our family and those around us. When the base chakra is in balance, we are able to function extremely well, we feel energized, adventurous, and vigorous, and we are good "providers", with a strong sense of loyalty to our family, community, and nation. But when imbalanced, we feel that life is a real struggle. There may be feelings of hopelessness as you strive to provide for yourself and your dependents, both physically and emotionally.

The sacral chakra: orange

The sacral chakra, located at the lower abdominal area, relates to reproductive disorders, the immune system, the bladder, the kidneys, the lower spine, and the hip and pelvic area, and vibrates at the same frequency as the colour orange.

This chakra is the centre from which we express ourselves and pour forth our creativity. In balance, it represents joy, spontaneity, and feelings of immense power. This is the area in which women carry and nourish their unborn babies. It has an affinity with feminine sexuality and the creation of life itself. When this chakra is in a state of imbalance, however, life can seem bleak and devoid of joy, and bringing forth creativity can seem like an impossible task, which is delegated to the mind, rather than left to the natural creative forces lying deep within us.

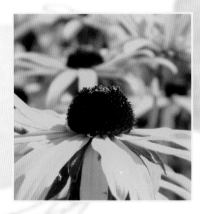

The solar plexus chakra: yellow

This chakra is also known as the "sun centre". It relates physically to the digestive organs, liver, gallbladder, and mid-back, and vibrates with the frequency of the colour yellow.

This is the centre of emotional intelligence, decision-making, and clarity. When working harmoniously, it is through the energy here that we form relationships, linking ourselves to our friends by means of energy cords. When this chakra is out of balance, however, we feel isolated from others, often finding it difficult to form and maintain long-term relation-ships, leading to loneliness.

The heart chakra: green

Resonating with the vibration of the colour green, this chakra is our centre of balance. Physically, it is associated with the heart and circulation, the lungs, shoulders, arms, as well as the ribs and breasts.

From this chakra, we are able to feel compassion and form loving relationships, being open and giving, both to ourselves and to others. With this energy, we learn to value ourselves, and we learn the gift of love. When this chakra is imbalanced, however, an excess or lack of green can lead to feelings of tightness, meanness, and jealousy toward others. We want to keep good things for ourselves and feel a reluctance to share. When this centre is very closed, it is impossible to have loving feelings, either toward ourselves or toward other people. We may even feel resentful of others' success, beauty, or good nature.

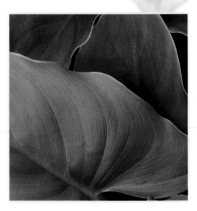

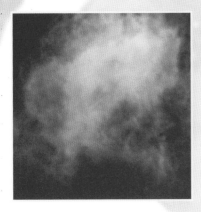

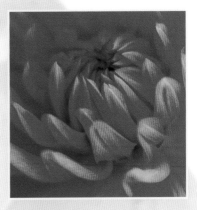

The third eye: violet

Situated between the eyebrows, this chakra vibrates at the same frequency as the colour violet. Physically, it is associated with the brain, the eyes, nose, and ears, as well as with the nervous system. It is called the "third eye" as it is the eye that looks within (rather than outwardly) for wisdom and knowledge.

The third eye chakra is the seat of everyone's feminine powers of insight and intuition – the energy that supports our instinctive "knowing" – and is connected to learning and the discerning acquisition of knowledge. It is with this energy that we can connect both with spiritual ideals and with the more mundane aspects of life, learning how to merge the two. An imbalance in this area can manifest as a "know-it-all" attitude. Life can then become over-intellectualized, potentially leading to an attitude that is domineering and overbearing.

The throat chakra: blue

This chakra supports the throat and neck vertebrae, the mouth, jaws, and teeth, and vibrates at the frequency of the colour blue.

From here, we are able to express ourselves with honesty and integrity. We are able to vocalize our thoughts and needs, and to follow our dreams honestly and with purity. We need this support to be in harmony in order for us to express truth. If the throat chakra becomes imbalanced in any way, it becomes impossible to voice our needs – even to ourselves. We tend to "choke back" our emotions, often feeling they are less important than the feelings of those around us, and we tend to defer to the authority of others.

The crown chakra: magenta

This chakra is located just above the crown of the head. The physical associations are with the skin, muscles, and skeletal system, and it vibrates with the same frequency as the colour magenta; although, it is also associated with white, which is the colour of spiritual growth and enlightenment. The same energy is thought to live within both magenta and white – it's just seen or experienced differently by different people.

Here, we discover our own deep spirituality, which is not concerned with dogma or organized religion. This is our personal growth, our personal connection with the Divine, and with all that is. An imbalance in this chakra can result in feelings of despair and worthlessness, where we seek, but do not find, the higher purpose – or a greater depth – in our existence. Life may seem superficial and meaningless.

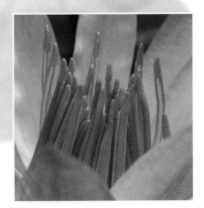

Chakra-balancing *exercise*

Spending a little time clearing and balancing ourselves energetically can work wonders in helping to prevent and alleviate migraines, as well as potentially giving us more insight into, and understanding of, the root of our symptoms.

There are few hard and fast rules about how to do this non-contact chakra "massage". You can do it on yourself or ask someone to do it for you. If you are working on a partner, you may use both hands at once. Many people feel more comfortable using the left hand to clear and the right hand to balance the chakra, but ultimately, the decision is yours. It is the direction in which you massage that is important as you are removing old, stagnant energy by working in a counterclock-wise direction and you are encouraging the energy centres to spin smoothly when working in a clockwise direction.

The length of time it takes to clear each chakra will vary according to its state of being at the time, but it generally takes two or three minutes to draw out old or toxic energy from each chakra. If, however, you feel that your energies are being disturbed too much, or you feel in any way uncomfortable, then it is advisable to start in the clock-wise direction straight away.

Occasionally, someone will experience a headachy feeling as the chakras are being worked on. This will usually disappear as you work your way up the body, as it is simply an indication that stale or toxic vibrations are being released and are travelling up the spine. If you already have a headache when you start this process, then try working from the crown of the head downward.

1 Lie down on your back on the floor, making sure that you will be warm enough, as the body has the tendency to become chilled when relaxing.

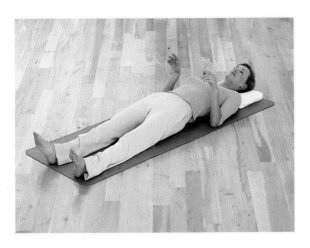

2 *Shake your hands to remove any surplus energy.*

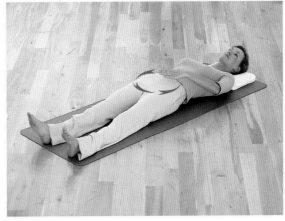

3 *Beginning with the base chakra, circle your hand in a counter-clockwise direction (to the left) above the surface of the body. There is no need to make contact with the skin as you are massaging your energy field only. Make your circles about the width of your body. You may feel a tingling feeling or heaviness in your hand as you gather old energy, so shake the hand to remove this.*

4 *Next, begin circling above the same chakra in a clockwise direction, winding in new energy and harmonizing and rebalancing yourself. You can use the opposite hand from step 3 if you wish.*

Move up the body and circle in a similar way through all the chakras, first clearing away old energy with one hand in a counterclockwise direction, and then introducing new energy with the other hand in a clockwise direction.

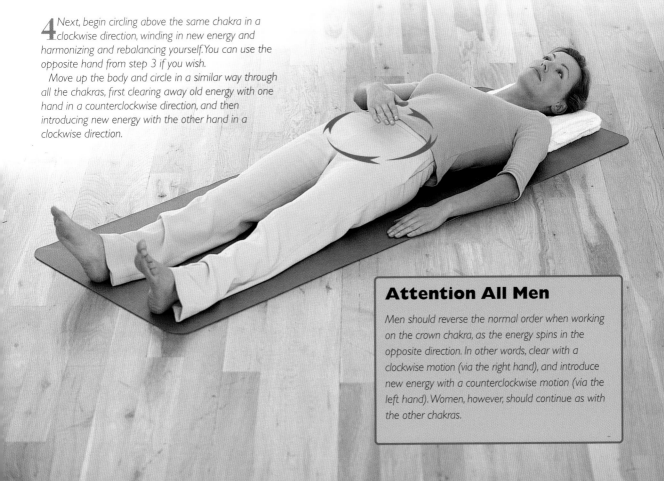

Attention All Men

Men should reverse the normal order when working on the crown chakra, as the energy spins in the opposite direction. In other words, clear with a clockwise motion (via the right hand), and introduce new energy with a counterclockwise motion (via the left hand). Women, however, should continue as with the other chakras.

Colour contemplation

The mind often becomes cluttered and over-concerned with trivia, which can lead to an overloaded mind and migraines. Colour visualization is a powerful way to help clear it of such unwanted thoughts and to bring added depth to contemplation.

Even if you cannot "see" colour, it is all around us in our energy fields. Whether or not you feel that you can see colour in your mind's eye, the following exercise can be of great value; by using the mind to create intention, you can still activate colours in your aura.

Read the section on chakras and their related colours on pages 115–117 to decide which colour you feel the need to work with. If you feel confused about which colour to use, then work with white as this contains all the colours of the spectrum.

This contemplation is great to do at any time, but particularly when in the throes of a debilitating migraine attack.

The exercise is made stronger if you make the effort to find an object from nature that displays your chosen colour – perhaps a flower, a plant, a gemstone, or a piece of fruit. Using this as a point of focus will help you look inside yourself within the context of nature's beauty, thus encouraging your energy to flow more harmoniously.

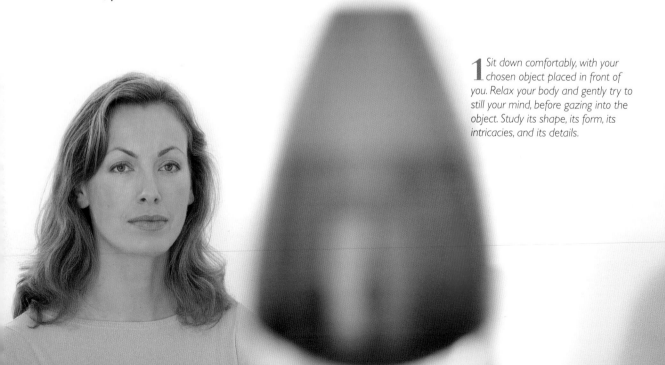

1 Sit down comfortably, with your chosen object placed in front of you. Relax your body and gently try to still your mind, before gazing into the object. Study its shape, its form, its intricacies, and its details.

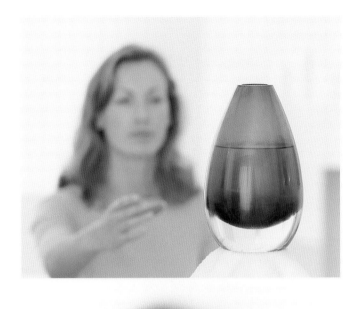

2 Reach toward your coloured object with your hands, trying to feel the vibration of the colour radiating from it.

3 Close your eyes and now just visualize your object in your mind, expanding it until you are aware only of its colour. As you breathe in, feel the colour filling your body, and as you breathe out, let it flood outward into your aura.

Take your attention to your headache, or what you perceive to be the cause of your headache, and focus into it. Gently breathe your colour into this pain, relaxing fully as you do so. Allow the gentle colour vibrations to wash away the pain and enjoy the feeling of relief and well-being.

You will know when the time is right to open your eyes and have a gentle stretch. Feel for any changes that may have taken place. You may experience a sense of greater clarity and peace, or your body may feel somehow lighter and less cluttered. Be patient with yourself, however, as it often takes a little practice for this exercise to become effective.

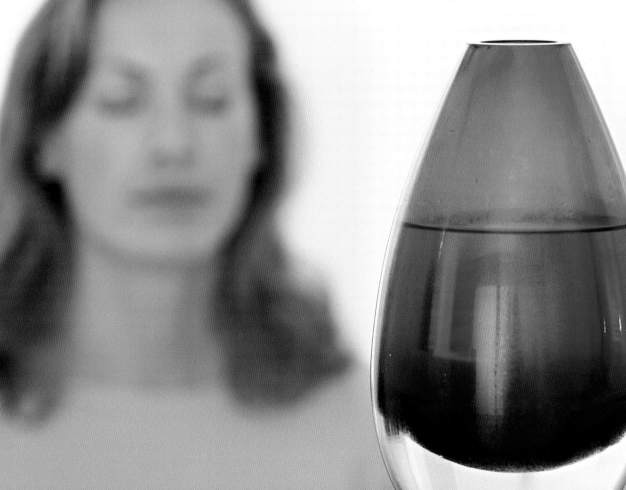

Colour-balancing *meditation*

This meditation takes a degree of practice for it to be of real benefit, but you will enjoy a greater sense of health and well-being afterwards. The purpose is to rebalance the body, mind, and spirit – it is particularly beneficial to relieve migraine pain.

Set aside at least ten minutes for yourself to do this exercise every now and again or when you feel a migraine coming on.

★ Lie down somewhere warm and comfortable. Systematically work through your body from the feet upward, tensing the muscles and then relaxing them, until your whole body feels relaxed and peaceful.

★ Take your awareness down to your base chakra, at the tip of your tail bone, and imagine that you are able to breathe deeply into this area. Then visualize that you are breathing in the colour red with each inhalation and releasing old or stagnant energy from this chakra with each exhalation. Become aware of your magnetic connection with the earth. Continue until the base chakra feels open and unblocked and the energy you

are breathing out feels as pure as the energy you are breathing in. Be aware of your aura filling with this wonderful, vibrant, energizing red.

★ Take your awareness up to the next chakra, located around the navel area, which is the sacral centre. Bring the colour orange into your awareness. Imagine, or intend, that you are breathing in the colour orange with each inhalation and breathing away unwanted energy with each exhalation. Continue until this chakra feels vibrant and open, and is radiating a glorious, warm orange into your aura – the energy of pure creative flow. Feel your connection with the creative flow of the universe.

★ Move your attention up to your solar plexus chakra, located around the top of the stomach. Visualize the bright yellow of the

summer sun coming into this area, like a beam of light. Absorb the joyous colour into your body as you breathe in and release it into your energy field as you breathe out. Feel your solar plexus relaxing and expanding as it resonates with yellow. Enjoy the feeling of clarity it brings. Allow any sludgy or stale energy

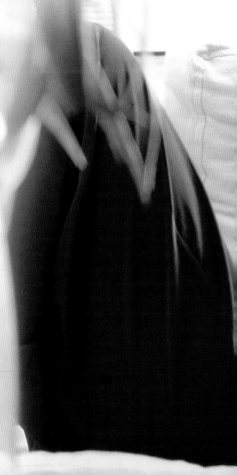

to sink away into the earth.
★ Moving upward to the heart chakra, now bring the colour green to mind – the fresh green of a spring morning. As you breathe in this colour, become aware of allowing your heart to relax and expand, letting any restrictions flow away. As you breathe green into your heart chakra, know that the vibration of this colour represents the harmony of natural forces. Allow these forces of nature to flood through your being, in the knowledge that you are part of the great flow of life.
★ Now bring your awareness to the throat chakra and the colour blue – the fresh blue of a clear summer sky. Absorb this gentle blue energy into your body and release it into your energy field. Breathe in new life and breathe

out old ways. Feel the throat chakra releasing and opening as it floods with the blue vibration.
★ Take your awareness up to the space between the eyebrows, the third eye, and bring the colour violet to mind. It may help to gently massage this area with slow, circular movements of the fingers as you begin to breathe in the colour. Imagine your third eye opening to let the colour in and your vision clearing. Breathe out any feelings of haziness or lack of vision, and feel yourself awakening to a greater reality. Allow the colour violet to gently permeate your aura.
★ Finally, take your awareness to the top of your head, to your crown chakra. Bring to mind the colour magenta. Breathe into the wisdom

contained within this colour, as the vibration of magenta brings a connection with the higher spiritual realms. Feel the opening of your crown chakra as you breathe in and release any old prejudices and limitations as you breathe out. Feel at one with all that is. When it feels right to do so, release this beautiful colour into your aura.
★ Relax and become aware of all the vibrations and colours that are now flowing and blending harmoniously around and throughout your being, playing out the glorious dance of life.

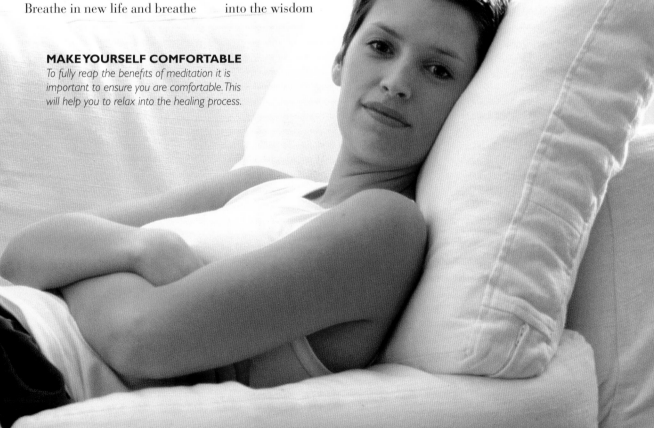

MAKE YOURSELF COMFORTABLE
To fully reap the benefits of meditation it is important to ensure you are comfortable. This will help you to relax into the healing process.

The power of blue

As you become more familiar with working internally with energy and colour, you may be able to start visualizing your migraines as certain negative colours in your mind's eye. This powerful exercise will help you transform these negative colours and energy forces into positive ones, thus lessening, or maybe even ridding you, of migraine-related pain.

Your migraine may, for instance, appear as a tense angry red at times of a throbbing headache, a dirtyish yellow in the case of a nauseous migraine, or a smudgy green in the case of a headache caused by emotional distress.

In all these instances – and all others – visualizing a beautiful, deep, refreshing blue in place of the previous negative colour will help alleviate the migraine symptoms by clearing stagnant energy.

Why blue?

Blue is a calming, contemplative colour, which brings an energy of peace and clarity. Our associations with the colour blue are often positive ones: a cloudless sky on a sunny day, a peaceful, slightly rippling lake, the lapping waves of the ocean – all symbolic of trusting and letting things flow and take their natural course – just as this book encourages you to do in order to release yourself from the destructive cycle of worry and stress that may be causing your migraines.

Lavender or pale violet is also a soothing, healing colour for the mind, and particularly good in alleviating migraines, so you could sometimes try this same exercise with the colour violet.

★ Sit cross-legged on the floor or on a chair or lie on your back on the floor – whatever is a comfortable, relaxing position for you.

★ Try to tune into and visualize what colour your migraine and its associated discomfort might be. Imagine yourself, and particularly your head, enveloped in this colour, restrained by it.

★ Then breathe a deep, rich blue into your body. Visualize yourself gradually filling up with this colour instead of the old one. If you find it difficult to visualize, simply intend it to be so. Allow the colour blue to flood through you, releasing and washing away the pain and discomfort of the previous colour related to your migraine attacks.

★ Feel the crown of your head relaxing more and more as the pain releases from your body – simply have the intention of letting it go. An increased sense of calm should come over you.

★ When you are ready, complete the process by allowing a gentle shower of white or rose-pink to wash through you from the crown of the head downward, cleansing away all blockages, old energy, and imbalances.

★ Then open your eyes, ready to face the world with renewed feelings of calm, health, and well-being, brought about by the release from the pain of headaches and migraines.

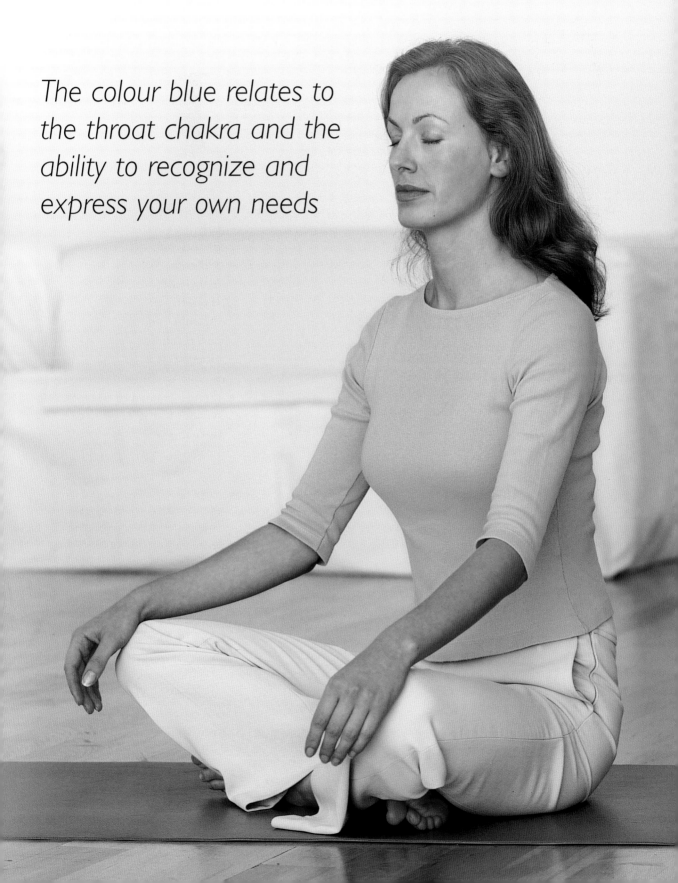

The colour blue relates to the throat chakra and the ability to recognize and express your own needs

Acknowledgements

A huge, heartfelt thanks to all the people who have had a hand in the writing and publishing of this book. The first thank you must go to my wonderful husband, Pete, for his unswerving help and support, to my much-loved children – Henry, Emily and Lucy – and to my very special parents, all of whom have been a huge inspiration to me in more ways than they will ever know. Also to Steve and Jane, who are so special and always seem to believe in me.

Thank you, too, to my enduring and inspired editor, Kelly, with whom I have shared many sleepless nights at the computer. A big thank you to all my patient friends who supported and encouraged me when I have been too busy to spend time with them. Thanks also go out to Helen – a great and gifted healer – who told me that I was "worth something" and gave me the momentum to turn my world around and follow my heart's desire. And finally, thank you to my clients, who have all been teachers to me, as well as dear friends. My hope is that everyone who reads this book will proceed further along their path toward healing and awareness. We all have our unique story to tell and our own journey to take, so enjoy your journey and the telling of your tale.